Soil and Greenhouse Effect
Monitoring and Mitigation

Soil and Greenhouse Effect

Monitoring and Mitigation

Editors

Dr. H. Pathak
M.Sc., Ph.D.
Senior Scientist, Division of Environmental Sciences,
Indian Agricultural Research Institute, New Delhi

and

Dr. S. Kumar
M.Sc., Ph.D.
Principal Scientist and Former Head,
Division of Environmental Sciences,
Indian Agricultural Research Institute, New Delhi

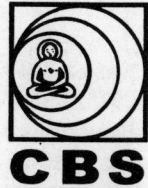

C B S

CBS PUBLISHERS & DISTRIBUTORS

NEW DELHI • BANGALORE

ISBN : 81-239-1040-1

First Edition : 2003
Reprint : 2008

Publishing Director : Vinod K. Jain

Published by :
Satish Kumar Jain for CBS Publishers & Distributors,
4819/XI, 24 Ansari Road, Darya Ganj, New Delhi - 110 002
E-mail : cbspubs@vsnl.com • Website : www.cbspd.com

Branch Office :
2975, 17th Cross, K.R. Road,
Bansankari 2nd Stage, Bangalore - 560 070
Fax : 080-26771680 • E-mail : cbsbng@vsnl.net

Printed at :
Asia Printograph, Shahdara, Delhi-110 032

Preface

THE EMISSION OF greenhouse gases to the atmosphere has become a matter of great concern because of the future projections of global warming and climate change. The greenhouse gases, viz. carbon dioxide, methane, and nitrous oxide in the atmosphere increase the global temperature due to the transmission of the incoming short-wave radiations and absorbence of the outgoing long-wave radiations. Agricultural soils contribute substantially to the greenhouse effect, primarily through the emission and consumption of these gases. From last two decades the research efforts have been intensified, particularly in the developing countries, on the quantitative measurement of emission of greenhouse gases from soil. As a result very useful information has been generated which has enriched our understanding on emission of these gases from soil under various land-use types.

Greenhouse effect and climate change have been included in the course curricula at school and university levels as a subject for teaching. The objective of preparing this book is to understand the processes and factors responsible for the formation and emission of these gases from soil and to take a stock of the mass of available information, summarize it and present it in a simple form to catalyze the practical application. The techniques for the measurement of greenhouse gas emission from soil have been illustrated and various mitigation options to reduce the emission of these gases have been suggested. Attempts have been made to identify the missing links and gaps in our information. The book, therefore, will serve the need of students, researchers, and policy makers.

The book would not have been the light of the day without the help and cooperation of our esteemed colleagues and friends, who have expertise in different aspects of greenhouse gas emission from soil and contributed different chapters of the book. We express our sincere gratitude and heartfelt thanks to each one of them.

Our colleagues and students at Indian Agricultural Research Institute,

New Delhi have contributed immensely for the preparation of the book. We take this opportunity to offer our sincere thanks and gratitude to Dr. P.K. Aggarwal, Dr. H.C. Joshi, Ms. Nimisha Srivastava, Dr. D. Majumdar, Dr. D.R. Biswas, Dr. Subhash Chander, Dr. S.D. Singh, Dr. R. Choudhury, Dr. Jagpal Singh, Mr. Sujith Kumar, Mr. Vinod Kumar, Mr. Pargat Singh, Mr. Pawan Kumar and Mrs. Sumita Pathak for their help and suggestions in preparing this book. We are thankful to Dr. B.S. Aggarwal, Ex-scientist, Council of Scientific and Industrial Research, New Delhi for meticulously going through manuscript and English editing. We thank Mr. S.K. Jain, Managing Director and Mr. H.S. Poplai, General Manager, CBS Publishers and Distributors, CBS PLAZA, 4819/11, Prahlad Street, 24 Ansari Road, Darya Ganj, New Delhi 110 002 for taking the responsibility of publishing the book.

We hope that we have been able to contribute towards a better understanding of the processes involved in the emission of greenhouse gases from soil, their monitoring and mitigation options. We shall deem our efforts successful if the book is proved useful to those for whom it is meant. Comments from the readers will help us to improve the book in future.

H. PATHAK
S. KUMAR

Foreword

OVER THE PAST few decades, the man-induced changes in the climate of the earth have become the focus of scientific and social attention. The most imminent of these is the increased levels of carbon dioxide and other greenhouse gases in the atmosphere leading to global warming. The 1990s was, on an average, the warmest decade of the earth since instrumental measurement of temperature started in 1860s and the 1900s the warmest century during the last 1000 years. Besides increase in temperature, the quantity of rainfall and its events has also become more uncertain. In certain places, climatic extremes such as droughts, floods, rainfall distribution and snowmelt have increased.

Alarmed by the possible adverse impact that the global climate change might have on the quality of life of human beings, there has been a serious concern all over the world in understanding the vulnerability of various regions and in developing strategies to mitigate the negative effects. These changes could considerably affect the food supply and access through their direct and indirect effects on crops, soils, livestock, fisheries and pests.

The Inter-Governmental Panel on Climatic Change (IPCC) of the United Nations in its recent report produced by more than 400 scientific experts has again confirmed the increasingly strong evidence for humanity's influence on the global climate and projected that the globally averaged temperature of the air above the earth's surface would rise by 1.4-5.8 degrees Celsius over the next 100 years. It has provided further evidence of the scale and seriousness of the global warming problem and need to act quickly and decisively.

Reduction of greenhouse gases emissions by decreasing fossil fuel combustions and other resource conservation measures can reduce global warming. Different countries under the umbrella of UN organizations are now intensively discussing the mitigation aspects. Developed countries have been in the forefront of this concern and have strengthened their research capacity to understand the greenhouse gases emissions from different sectors and regions, and their mitigation options.

The trade-off of such reductions with development, income and overall quality of human life is, however, forcing many such countries not to implement the mitigation strategies and to shift the emphasis of emission control to the developing world. Methane emission from rice paddies is a typical example. The research of the western world concluded that rice paddies of Asia emit large amount of methane, a greenhouse gas with larger warming potential than even CO_2. Systematic studies done in our country later helped in changing the opinion. In global policy negotiations, where different pressure groups force adoption of international policy measures that could have a differential impact on different parts of the world, negotiators of our own country as well as many other developing countries look forward to indigenous research backups. This book by Pathak and Kumar of the Division of Environmental Sciences, Indian Agricultural Research Institute, on greenhouse gases emission from agricultural soils, is, therefore, very timely and welcome addition.

The subject of greenhouse emission has now been included in the course curricula of the discipline of environmental sciences at school and university levels all over the country. The need of a text-book on greenhouse gas emission from agriculture has been felt for sometime. This book deals with the processes of greenhouse effect, global warming; emissions, measurement techniques and mitigation of greenhouse gas emissions from soil as well as impact on Indian agriculture. The glossary of terms frequently used and bibliography will be of particular interest to the students.

I appreciate the efforts put by the editors and the authors in collecting the available information and bringing out the book and hope this will be very useful for the students, researchers and policy makers working in the field of global climate change and agriculture.

December 30, 2002

(P.K. AGGARWAL)
Head
Division of Environmental Sciences
Indian Agricultural Research Institute
New Delhi 110 012

List of contributors

Ms. Banerjee, Bidisha, Scientist, Division of Environmental Sciences, Indian Agricultural Research Institute, New Delhi 110 012

Dr. Bhatia, Arti, Scientist, Division of Environmental Sciences, Indian Agricultural Research Institute, New Delhi 110 012

Dr. Chatterjee, A., Senior Research Fellow, Division of Environmental Sciences, Indian Agricultural Research Institute, New Delhi 110 012

Dr. Chaudhary, Anita, Senior Scientist, Division of Environmental Sciences, Indian Agricultural Research Institute, New Delhi 110 012

Mr. Govind, A., Research Scholar, Division of Agricultural Physics, Indian Agricultural Research Institute, New Delhi 110 012

Dr. Jain, M. C., Former Head, Division of Environmental Sciences, Indian Agricultural Research Institute, New Delhi 110 012

Dr. Jain, Niveta, Scientist, Division of Environmental Sciences, Indian Agricultural Research Institute, New Delhi 110 012

Ms. Jyothi Kumari, Research Scholar, Division of Soil Science and Agricultural Chemistry, Indian Agricultural Research Institute, New Delhi 110 012

Dr. Kalra, N., Principal Scientist and Head, Unit for Applications of Systems Simulation, Indian Agricultural Research Institute, New Delhi 110 012

Dr. Kumar, S., Former Head, Division of Environmental Sciences, Indian Agricultural Research Institute, New Delhi 110 012

Ms. Mazumdar, Sonali, Research Scholar, Division of Soil Science and Agricultural Chemistry, Indian Agricultural Research Institute, New Delhi 110 012

Dr. Mitra, S., Research Fellow, University of Bonn, Germany

Dr. Pathak, H., Senior Scientist, Division of Environmental Sciences, Indian Agricultural Research Institute, New Delhi 110 012

Mr. Prasad, S., Scientist, Division of Environmental Sciences, Indian Agricultural Research Institute, New Delhi 110 012

Mr. Puri, S., Senior Research Fellow, Division of Environmental Sciences, Indian Agricultural Research Institute, New Delhi 110 012

Dr. Rai, H.K., Research Associate, Division of Environmental Sciences, Indian Agricultural Research Institute, New Delhi 110 012

Mr. Sharma, A.K., Senior Research Fellow, Division of Environmental Sciences, Indian Agricultural Research Institute, New Delhi 110 012

Mr. Sharma, V., Senior Research Fellow, Division of Environmental Sciences, Indian Agricultural Research Institute, New Delhi 110 012

Mr. Singh, P.K., Senior Research Fellow, Division of Environmental Sciences, Indian Agricultural Research Institute, New Delhi 110 012

Mr. Singh, R., Research Scholar, Division of Environmental Sciences, Indian Agricultural Research Institute, New Delhi 110 012

Mr. Soni, U.A., Research Associate, Division of Environmental Sciences, Indian Agricultural Research Institute, New Delhi 110 012

Contents

Preface *v*
Foreward *vii*
List of contributors *ix*
List of abbreviations *xii*

1. Soil and greenhouse effect **1**
   H. Pathak and S. Kumar
2. Emission of methane from soil **18**
   H. Pathak, S. Kumar, Niveta Jain and S. Mitra
3. Nitrous oxide emission from soil **33**
   H. Pathak, Arti Bhatia, S. Prasad and V. Sharma
4. Carbon dioxide emission from soil **47**
   H. Pathak, Monika Rastogi, H.K. Rai and Anil Sharma
5. Ammonia volatilization from soil **56**
   H. Pathak, Bidisha Banerjee and Sonali Mazumdar
6. Measurement of greenhouse gas emission from soil and developing emission inventories **65**
   M.C. Jain, H. Pathak and Arti Bhatia
7. Global warming and soil microbial activity **79**
   Anita Chaudhary, S. Puri, N. Kalra and H. Pathak
8. Impact of climate change on Indian agriculture **86**
   A. Chatterjee, H. Pathak, U.A. Soni and N. Kalra
9. Carbon sequestration in soil **96**
   S. Mazumdar, B. Banerjee, R. Singh and H. Pathak
10. Mitigation of nitrous oxide emission from soil **106**
    H. Pathak, V. Sharma, Arti Bhatia and P. K. Singh
11. International initiatives on combating global warming **115**
    Jyothi Kumari, A. Govind and H. Pathak

Glossary **125**
Bibliography **139**
Subject Index **149**
Author Index **155**

List of abbreviations

BNF	Biological nitrogen fixation	MAC	Methane Asia Campaign
CEC	Cation exchange capacity	N	Nitrogen
CH_4	Methane	N_2O	Nitrous oxide
CO_2	Carbon dioxide	N_2O-N	N_2O calculated as amount
DAP	Diammonium phosphate		of N
DCD	Dicyandiamide	NATP	National Agricultural
DST	Department of Science and		Technology Project of
	Technology		ICAR
ECD	Electron capture detector	NCU	Neem coated urea
Eh	Redox potential	NH_3	Ammonia
FID	Flame ionization detector	NH_4^+-N	NH_4^+ as amount of N
FYM	Farmyard manure	NO_3-N	NO_3^- as amount of N
GC	Gas chromatograph	PET	Potential evapotranspira-
GCM	General Circulation Models		tion
Gg	Giga gram (10^9 g)	ppm	Parts per million
GM	Green manure	Pg	Peta gram (10^{15} gram)
Gt	Giga ton (10^9 ton)	SOC	Soil organic carbon
GWP	Global warming potential	SOM	Soil organic matter
IARI	Indian Agricultural	Tg	Tera gram (10^{12} g)
	Research Institute	UNEP	United Nations
ICAR	Indian Council of		Environment Programme
	Agricultural Research	USEPA	United State Environment
IPCC	Inter-Governmental Panel		Protection Agency
	on Climate Change	USG	Urea super granule
IRRI	International Rice	UV-	Ultra violet radiations
	Research Institute	radiations	

CHAPTER 1

Soil and greenhouse effect

H. PATHAK *and* S. KUMAR

*"The earth is a generous mother, she will provide in plentiful
abundance food for all her children if they will but cultivate her
soil in justice and in peace." — Bourke Cockran*

SOIL IS A NATURAL resource and can be defined as a "mass of inorganic material that holds inorganic and organic colloids, dead and living plant and animal material, water and gases in variable but balanced proportions". Long ago, Aristotle visualized soil as the 'source of infinite life'. The Chinese saying, 'the soil is the mother of all things' underlines the importance of soil to life of all living creatures. Currently, over 90% of the world food comes from the soil and less than 10% comes from water, both inland and the oceans. As the world soil resources are finite, intensive land-use is inevitable to meet the global demands for food and fibre. On the other hand, there are concerns worldover about sustainability arising due to decreasing soil productivity. Today the management of soil is, therefore, very important for development as we are crossing the threshold of new land available for cultivation.

Climate influences plant life in many ways and can inhibit, stimulate, alter or modify crop performance. Its components—temperature, solar radiation, rainfall, relative humidity and wind velocity—independently or in combination influence crop growth and productivity. All over the world concern has been expressed about the possible climate change caused by the increase in the concentration of greenhouse gases in the atmosphere. This threat of climate change has emerged as the most prominent global environment issue. Though the gravity of the threat and its implications are perceived differently by different people, there is no doubt that the concentrations of the greenhouse gases in the atmosphere are increasing of late at an alarming rate and there is undoubted international agreement that this increase in concentration of greenhouse gases will cause global warming and climate change. Using General Circulation Models (GCMs), it has been predicted that the doubling of the current carbon dioxide (CO_2) level in the atmosphere will cause an increase of 1.5 to 4.0 °C in average global surface air temperature, with accompanying changes in rainfall pattern by the end of the 21st century (Adams *et al.*, 1995). A similar increase has been predicted for the Indian subcontinent also (Sinha and Swaminathan, 1991). Although the solar radiation received at the surface will be variable geographically, on an average it is expected to decrease by about 10% (Hume and Cattle, 1990). In this chapter, we will discuss about the mechanism of greenhouse effect and global warming, the major greenhouse gases, the impact of global warming, estimates of greenhouse gas emission from agriculture and the strategies to reduce the greenhouse gas emission from agriculture.

GREENHOUSE EFFECT AND GLOBAL WARMING

Global warming is defined as the increase in the temperature of globe due to transmission of incoming short-wave radiation from the sun and the absorbency of outgoing long-wave radiation from the earth. This has been aggravated by the building up of some gases viz., carbon dioxide (CO_2), methane (CH_4), nitrous oxide (N_2O) and chlorofluoro carbons (CFCs). These are collectively called as greenhouse gases and they inhibit the outgoing radiations from the earth and upset earth's heat balance. The phenomenon is called 'Greenhouse Effect'. In the ordinary usage it simply means that the average air temperature will increase as a result of the build up of greenhouse gases in the atmosphere. Such global warming has been under way already for some time and is largely responsible for the temperature increase of the atmosphere by about 1°C that has occurred since 1860 (Figure 1).

Due to the greenhouse effect, warming of the lower atmosphere and surface of a planet takes place by a complex process involving sunlight, gases and particles in the atmosphere (Figure 2). All bodies absorb as well as transmit energy. The absorption may be over the whole range of wavelengths or it may be concentrated in one or more bands of wavelength. Radiations from the sun and earth closely resemble blackbody radiations. The radiation intensity increases with rise in temperature; the latter is a measurement of heat energy of a body. The higher the temperature, the lesser is the wavelength. For the sun that has an average temperature of about 6000°C, this wavelength is close to 0.5 micrometre. The earth's surface radiates most intensely near 10 micrometres at a mean surface temperature of 15°C. Greenhouse gases in the air can temporarily absorb thermal infra-red light of specific wavelengths and so not all the infra-red radiations

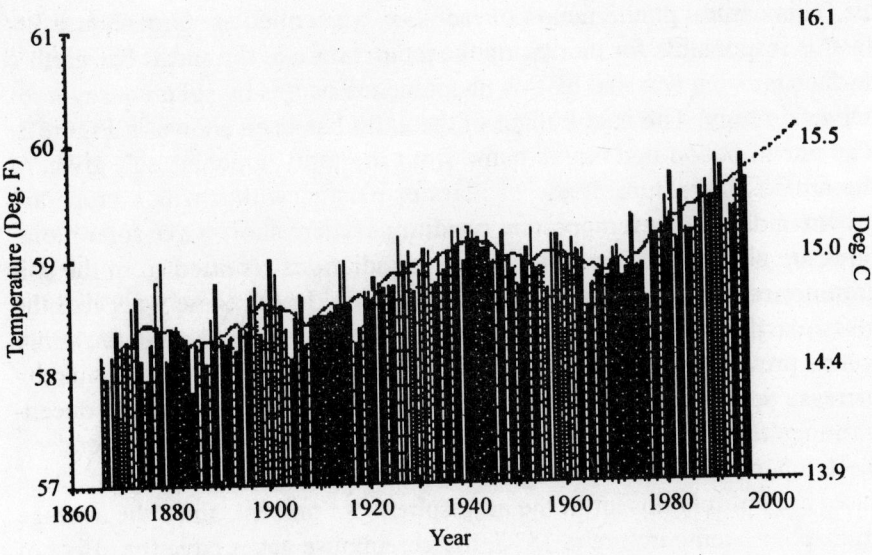

Figure 1: Rise of temperature with time (IPCC, 1996).

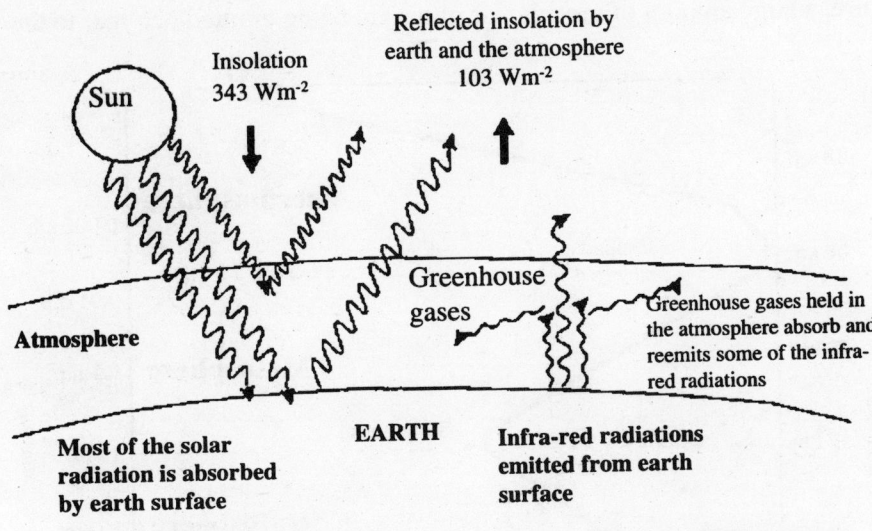

Figure 2: Global warming by greenhouse gases—A schematic representation.

emitted from the earth's surface escape directly into space from the atmosphere. Shortly after its absorption by the molecules in the atmosphere, this infrared light is re-emitted in all directions—completely randomly. Thus, some thermal infra-red radiations redirected back to earth's surface, are reabsorbed and consequently, further warms both the surface and the air. This natural phenomenon of radiation trap called as 'Greenhouse Effect' is responsible for increasing the temperature of the earth. The earth's surface is much warmed by this phenomenon as it is by solar energy it receives directly. The heat budget of the earth has been shown in Figure 3. The phenomenon derives its name from the term 'greenhouse', given to the artificial structure, made of glass or plastic, within which crops are grown under higher temperature conditions where short-wave solar radiations are allowed inside and long-wave radiations remitted from the soil are trapped to increase the temperature inside. In the same way, like the glass/plastic panels in the 'greenhouse', the greenhouse gases in the atmosphere prevent the escape of thermal radiations back to space and thereby increase the temperature of earth's atmosphere. Though the total concentration of the greenhouse gases in the atmosphere is less than one per cent, the temperature of the atmosphere becomes −18°C on average if these gases are entirely absent in the atmosphere. At present, since the average atmospheric temperature is 15°C, the greenhouse gases have the effect of warming the atmosphere from −18°C to 15°C, i.e., a rise of 33°C. On the earth, the greenhouse effect began long before human beings existed. However, with the advent of industrial revolution and intensive agriculture, a huge amount of greenhouse gases are being emitted per year to the

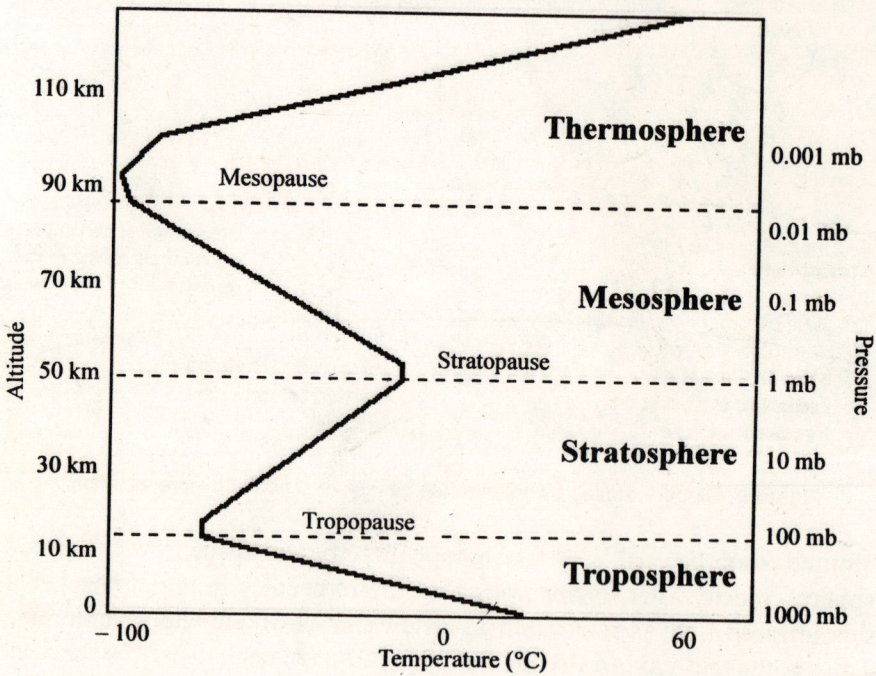

Figure 3: Structure of the atmosphere and change in temperature with altitude.

atmosphere due to industrial emissions, fossil fuel combustion, widespread deforestation, burning of biomass, as well as changes in land-use and land-management practices. The phenomenon that worries the scientists is that the increase in concentrations of the greenhouse gases in the atmosphere would increase the average surface temperature of the earth beyond 15 °C. This phenomenon has been termed as 'enhanced greenhouse effect' to distinguish its effects from the natural phenomenon of greenhouse effect that has been taking place for centuries.

OZONE LAYER DEPLETION

Most of the ozone in the atmosphere, the so-called "ozone layer", is in the lower stratosphere, at an altitude of about 20-25 kilometres above sea level (Figure 3). It acts as a shield by absorbing high-energy ultraviolet light (called UV-B) from the sun. If the ozone layer is depleted, more of these UV-B radiations reach the surface of the earth. Increased exposure to UV-B radiations has harmful effects on plants and animals, including humans causing skin cancer, eye damage and cataracts, and possible inhibition of immune system. Plants also suffer under increased UV-B radiations, and their vulnerability could result in reduced crop yields, damage to forest ecosystems, and decreased population of phytoplanktons in the world's oceans. The chemistry of ozone formation and destruction has been depicted in Figure 4.

Nitrous oxide, besides causing global warming, is responsible for the

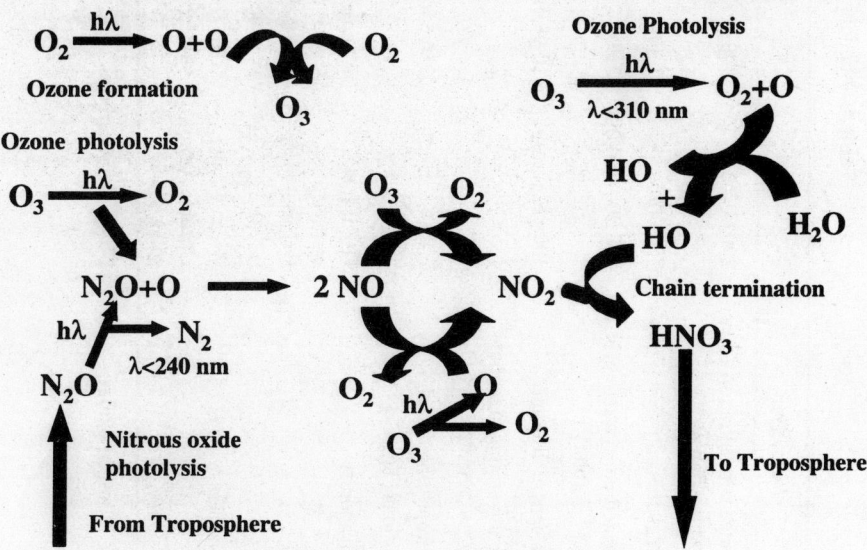

Figure 4: Chemistry of ozone in the stratosphere.

Table 1. Abundance, life-time and sources of greenhouse gases

Parameters	CO_2	CH_4	N_2O	NOx[†]	SO_2	$CFCs$[‡]
Average concentration 100 years ago (ppbV)	290,000	900	285	0.001-?	0.03-?	0
Current concentration (ppbV)	356,000	1,700	310	0.001-50	0.03-50	3
Projected concentration in the year 2030 (ppbV)	400,000-500,000	2,200-2,500	330-350	0.001-50	0.03-50	2.4-6
Atmospheric lifetime	100 years	10 years	166 years	Few days	Few weeks	75 years
Global warming potential (100 years relative to CO_2)	1	21	310	-	-	CFC11-4000 CFC12-8500
Anthropogenic/Total emissions (Tg yr^{-1})	5,500/ ~5,500	350/550	6/25	25/40	115/175	~1/1
Main sources	Fossil fuel combustion, Deforestation	Rice fields, Cattle, Landfills, Fossil-fuel combustion	Nitrogenous fertilizers, Deforestation, Biomass burning	Fossil fuel combustion, Biomass burning	Fossil fuel combustion, Ore smelting	Aerosol Sprays, Refrigerants, Foams
Main sinks	Green plants, Oceans, Atmospheric reactions	Removal in stratosphere, Soil	Oxidation in stratosphere	Oxidation in troposphere	Atmospheric reactions, Precipitation	Atmospheric reactions

[†]NOx, Nitrogen oxides;   [‡]CFCs, Chlorofluorocarbons

destruction of stratospheric ozone and also hinders the ozone forming 'Chapman reaction' in the stratosphere.

$$O + O_2 + M \longrightarrow O_3 + M \tag{i}$$

$$O_3 + O \longrightarrow 2O_2 \tag{ii}$$

When atomic and molecular oxygen collide, ozone is formed (Eq. i) and survives the collision provided that a third inert entity (M), normally N_2, is present in excess to absorb the energy.

Nitrous oxide reacts with the excited oxygen to form nitric oxide

$$N_2O + O \longrightarrow 2NO \tag{iii}$$

This reaction leads to reduction in the ozone formation, as atomic oxygen is not available for reacting with molecular oxygen to form ozone as shown in Eq. (i). Also nitric oxide formed from nitrous oxide leads to ozone decomposition:

$$NO + O_3 \longrightarrow NO_2 + O_2 \tag{iv}$$

GREENHOUSE GASES AND GLOBAL WARMING POTENTIAL

There are several gases that contribute to the greenhouse effect. Amongst them carbon dioxide is the most important, contributing 60% of global warming followed by methane (15%) and nitrous oxide (5%). The atmospheric abundance, life-time, sources and sinks of greenhouse gases are given in Table 1. During the past 250 years, the atmospheric concentrations of carbon dioxide, methane and nitrous oxide have increased by 30, 145 and 15%, respectively (Mosier *et al.*, 1998) but this increase has been more alarming during last 50 years (Figure 5). Though the atmospheric concentrations of the methane and nitrous oxide are much lower than that of carbon dioxide, their global warming potential is much higher. Global warming potential (GWP) is an index defined as the cumulative radiative forcing between the present and some chosen later time '*horizon*' caused by a unit mass of gas emitted now. It is used to compare the effectiveness of each greenhouse gas to trap heat in the atmosphere relative to some standard gas, by convention CO_2. The GWP for CH_4 (based on a 100-year time horizon) is 21, while that for N_2O, it is 310. Although present in lower concentrations than either CO_2 or CH_4, nitrous oxide is a very potent greenhouse gas, accounting for about 5 per cent of the enhanced greenhouse effect. By using global warming potential values for CH_4 and N_2O emissions as 21 and 310, respectively, we can convert all emission estimates to either a CO_2 or carbon equivalent (CE) base. Carbon dioxide equivalents can be calculated by multiplying the CE values by 3.7. Thus, the future global warming commitment of a greenhouse gas over the reference time horizon

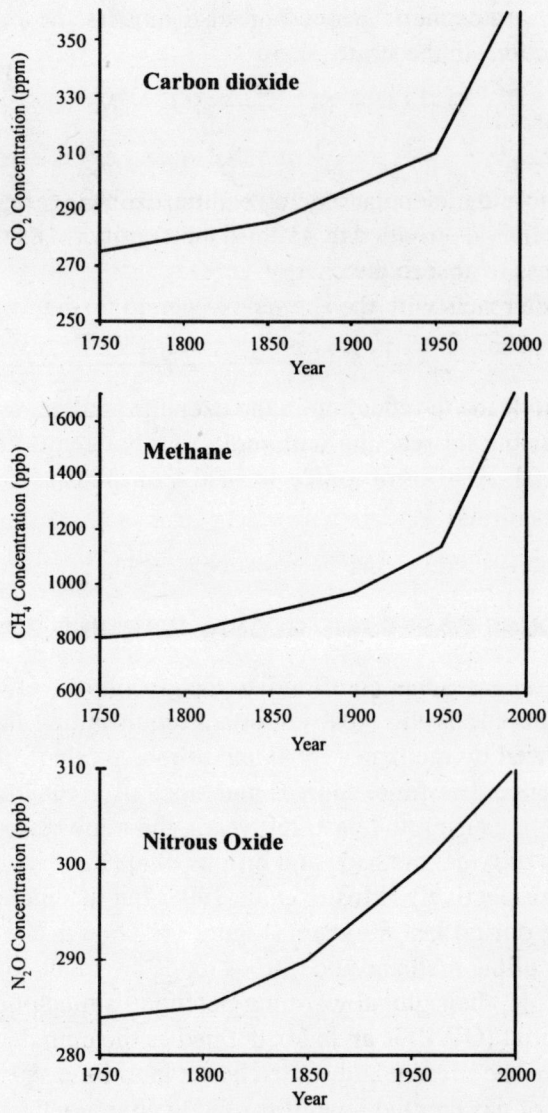

Figure 5: Rise in the concentration of greenhouse gases in the atmosphere.

is the appropriate global warming potential measured multiplied by the amount of gas emitted.

ENERGY ABSORPTION BY GREENHOUSE GASES

A gas absorbs light when the frequency of an internal motion within the gas molecule matches the frequency of the light that it encounters. For frequencies in the infrared region, the relevant motions are the vibrations of the molecule's atoms relative to each other. The simplest vibrational motion in a molecule is the oscillatory motion of the two bonded atoms X and Y relative to each other. In this motion, called band stretching, the distance between X and Y increases beyond its average value of R, then contracts to a lesser value, and finally returns to the original value of R. Such oscillatory motion occurs in all bonds of all molecules under all temperature conditions, even at absolute zero. A large number of such vibrational cycles occur each second. The exact frequency of the oscillatory motion depends primarily upon the type of bond, i.e. whether it is a single, double or triple bond, and upon the identity of the two atoms involved. For many bond types, for example, with the CH bond in methane and the CO bond in carbon monoxide, the stretching frequency does not fall in the thermal infra-red region. The stretching frequency of the carbon fluoride bonds does, however, fall within the thermal infrared range of 4-50 micrometre and thus molecules in the atmosphere with C—F bonds will absorb outgoing thermal infra-red light and enhance the greenhouse effect.

The other relevant type of vibration is an oscillation in the distance between two atoms X and Z bonded to a common atom Y, but not bonded to each other. Such motion alters the XYZ bond angle from its original value ϕ and is called angle bending vibration. All molecules containing three or more atoms possess bending vibrations. The oscillatory cycle of bond angle increases followed by a decrease and then another increase and so on. In order to absorb infra-red light, the molecule must have a dipole moment, i.e. there must be a difference in the position of the molecule between its centre of positive charge of the nuclei and the center of negative charge of its electron "cloud". These centres of charge coincide in free atoms and in homonuclear diatomic molecules like O_2 and N_2 and therefore, they do not absorb infra-red light. For CO_2, during the asymmetric stretch vibration when one CO bond contracts while the other expands or *vice versa*, the dipole moment of the molecule changes resulting in the absorption of the infra-red light.

IMPACT OF GREENHOUSE EFFECT

Greenhouse effect can lead to regional and global changes in climate and climate-related parameters such as temperature, rainfall, soil moisture, and sea level. Human health, terrestrial and aquatic ecological systems, agriculture, forestry, fisheries, and water resources are sensitive to changes in climate (Figure 6). According to the projections made in 1992 by the Inter-governmental Panel for Climate Change (IPCC, 1996), a group sponsored by the United Nations Environmental Programme, if no additional steps are taken to reduce emissions of CO_2 and the other problematic gases, then by the year 2040 the average global air temperature will be 1°C

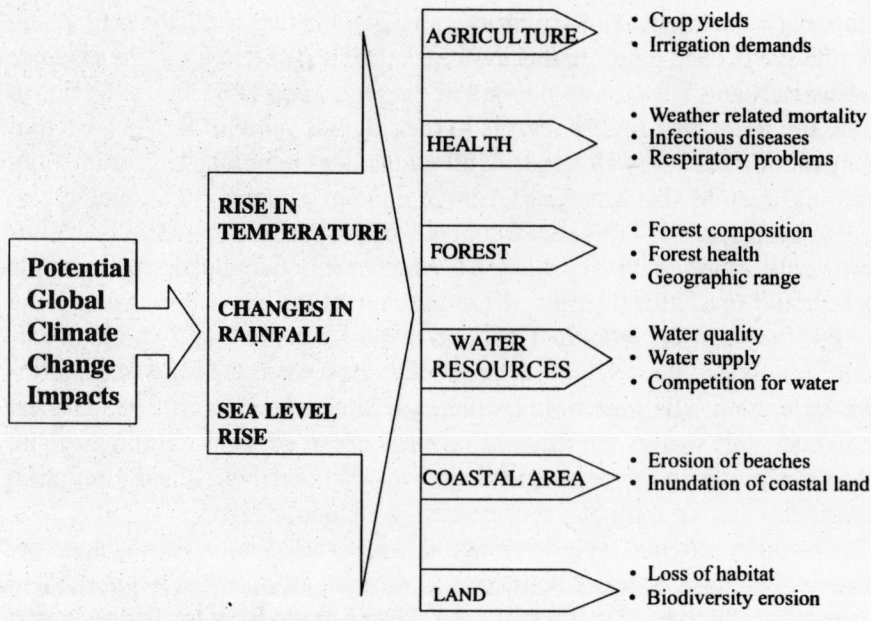

Figure 6: Possible impacts of climate change.

higher than at present. By 2100 it will increase still by 1.5°C. The temperature increase will probably be greater towards the Polar Regions. The total amount of global rainfall will increase, although there will be regions that will receive less and erratic rainfall than before these changes take place. Considering the usual scenario, CO_2 is projected to increase at the rate of 1.8 ppm per year reaching 397-416 ppm by 2010 and 605-755 by 2070 (Watson *et al.*, 1996). This along with changes in other greenhouse gases is likely to result in a temperature increase. How much will be the magnitude of climate change, where and in what time frame, remains uncertain. At the same time, there is an increased possibility of climate extremes such as the timings of onset of monsoon, intensities and frequencies of drought and floods.

Agriculture is sensitive to short-term changes in weather and to diurnal, seasonal, annual and long-term variations in climate. The climate elements, which affect the plant growth and development, hence the agriculture as a whole, are carbon dioxide concentration, temperature, radiation, precipitation and humidity. These are likely to be altered with the increased build up of greenhouse gases in the atmosphere and considerably affect the food supply and access through their direct and indirect effects on crops, soils, livestock, fisheries and pests. The increase in atmospheric CO_2 concentration promotes the growth and productivity of C3 plants. Increase in temperature, on the other hand, can reduce crop duration, enhance crop respiration rates, affect the equilibrium between crops and pests, hasten nutrient mineralization in soils, decrease fertilizer-use efficiencies, and increase evapotranspiration. Indirectly, there may be considerable impact on agricultural land-use due to snow melt, availability of irrigation, frequency and intensity of inter- and intra-seasonal droughts and floods, soil organic matter transformations, soil erosion, decline in arable areas (due to submergence of coastal lands), and availability of energy. All these changes would have tremendous impact on agricultural production and hence, food security of any region. Potential impact of climate change on agriculture is given below.

1. The climate change may reduce average crop yields and may lead to decreased yield stability. However, some plants may increase photosynthesis because of higher temperature and CO_2, but all plants will not be benefited.

2. The total amount of global rainfall will increase, although there will be regions that may receive less rainfall than before. The El-Nino effect, which invades world's oceans and continents every decade, is suggested to get a big boost by the rise in temperature of the atmosphere.

3. Demand for irrigation is likely to increase in all regions. It will lead to higher competition for existing water resources. Increase in temperature may also result in a higher amount of evapo-transpiration, which may lead to increased frequency of droughts and demand for irrigation.

4. Ranges and populations of agricultural pests currently limited by temperature may change. Higher temperature may increase diseases and heat stress. Some livestock diseases that are limited to tropical countries at present, such as Rift Valley fever and African swine fever, may spread, causing serious economic losses.

5. Sea levels will rise by about 18 cm by 2040 and by 48 cm by 2100, attributed mainly due to thermal expansion of water and melting of glaciers. Although this sea rise may look small but there are countries such as Bangladesh, Maldives, etc. where much of the population currently lives on the land that would be flooded by a sea level rise of just about 50 cm. Sea level rise could also affect fisheries directly and indirectly through the availability of feed.

6. Alteration of the energy balance and circulation system in the World Ocean will directly affect the productivity of the marine ecosystem.

7. Increase in temperature is likely to affect the crop calendars in low latitude regions, particularly where more than one crop is harvested in a year.

INTERDEPENDENCY OF SOIL AND CLIMATE CHANGE

Soil and climate change are related by bi-directional interactions (Figure 7). Practically all soil processes related to agriculture are directly affected in one way or the other by the climate. Changes in temperature and precipitation can influence soil water-content, runoff, erosion, salinization, biodiversity and organic carbon and nitrogen content. Changes in soil water induced by global climate change may affect all soil processes and ultimately the crop growth.

(a) Increase in temperature would cause more evapo-transpiration, which may result in lowering of groundwater table at some places.

(b) The increased temperature coupled with reduced rainfall may lead to upward water movement resulting in accumulation of salts in upper soil layers.

(c) Similarly, rise in sea level associated with increased temperature may lead to salt-water ingression in the coastal lands turning them unsuitable for conventional agriculture.

(d) Organic matter content, which is already quite low in most parts of the world, would become still lower and climatic change may affect its quality. Increase in atmospheric CO_2 concentration may compensate for increased decomposition of soil organic matter but the net balance would depend upon the carbon inputs and losses. There are reports that residues of crops under elevated CO_2 concentration have higher C:N ratio, and this may reduce their rate of decomposition in soils leading to an increment in ecosystem carbon stock.

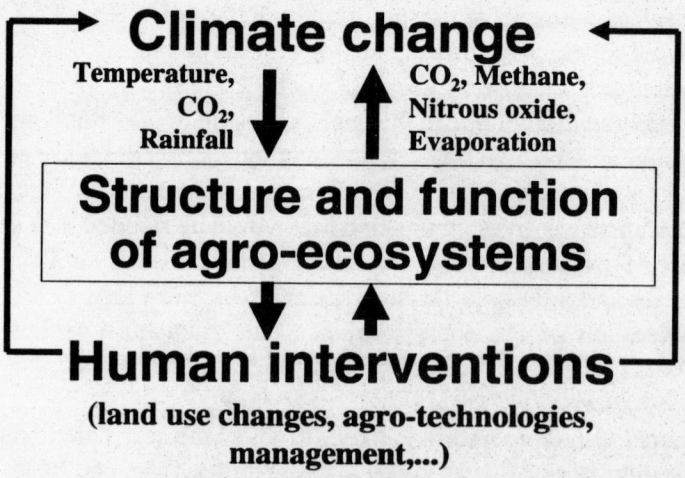

Figure 7: Interdependency of agriculture and climate change.

Table 2. Inventory of greenhouse gases in 1990 along with the relative contribution of agriculture to total emission...

Item	CO₂ (Tg)	CO₂ (% of the world)	CH₄ (Tg)	CH₄ (% of the world)	GWP of CH₄	% GW caused by CO₂	N₂O (Tg)	N₂O (% of the world)	GWP of N₂O	% GW caused by CO₂
World	26400	100	535	100	11235	42.6	9.0	100	2774.5	10.5
India	585	2.1	18.5	3.5	388.5	1.5	0.3	2.8	79.1	0.3
World Agriculture	—	—	167.5	31.3	3517.5	13.3	3.5	39.1	1085.0	4.1
Indian Agriculture	—	—	11.4	2.1	238.8	0.9	0.2	2.3	62.6	0.2
Enteric fermentation	—	—	7.3	1.4	153.3	0.6	0.0	0.1	3.4	0.0
Manure management	—	—	0.4	0.1	7.4	0.0	—	—	—	—
Agricultural soils	—	—	3.6	0.7	76.4	0.3	0.2	1.8	51.2	0.2
Burning of residues	—	—	0.1	0.0	1.8	0.0	0.0	0.3	8.1	0.0

GW, Global Warming; GWP, Global Warming Potential
Source: Watson *et al.* (1996), Garg and Shukla (2002)

Table 3. Options for the mitigation of greenhouse gas emissions from agriculture

Mitigation options	Mitigation potential†		
	CO_2	CH_4	N_2O
1. Land conversion and management			
— Reduced deforestation rate	H	M	M
— Pasture immediately after deforestation	M		L
— Conversion of marginal agricultural land to grassland, forest	M		L
2. Agricultural land utilization and management			
— Restoring productivity of degraded soils	H	L	
— More intensive use of existing farmlands	M	L	L
— Restricted use of organic soils	H		L
— Conservation tillage	M		L
— Reduction of dry land fallowing	M		
— Diversified rotations with forage crops	M		L
3. Biofuels			
— Energy crops for fossil fuel substitution	H		
— Agro-forestry	L		
— Windbreaks and shelter belts	L		
— Agro-industrial wastes for fossil fuel substitution	L		
4. Rice cropping systems			
— Irrigation management		M	L
— Nutrient management		M	L
— New cultivars		M	L
5. Plant nutrient management			
— Improved fertilizer-use efficiency	L		H
— Nitrification inhibitors			M
— Legume cropping to booster system productivity			M
— Integrating crop and animal farming			L
6. Recycling of livestock and other wastes			
— Recycling of municipal organic wastes	L	L	M
— Biogas production from manure		M	

†H, high; M, medium; L, low
Source: IPCC (1996)

(e) Increase of soil temperature by 1 °C may help in increased mineralization but N-availability for crop growth may still decrease due to increased gaseous losses through processes such as volatilization.

(f) Biological nitrogen fixation under elevated concentrations of CO_2 may show an increase, provided other nutrients are not limiting.

(g) The change in rainfall volume and frequency, and wind may alter the severity, frequency and extent of soil erosion.

These changes may further compound the direct effect of temperature and CO_2 on crop growth and yield. All these effects, however, would be highly region specific, depending upon the magnitude of climatic change, basic soil properties and current climatic conditions.

Soil is considered to be one of the most important sources and sinks of greenhouse gases, thus directly influencing climate change and indirectly through the production and consumption of ammonia (NH_3), nitrogen oxides (NOx) and carbon monoxide (CO). It contributes about 20% to the total emission of carbon dioxide through soil respiration and root respiration, 12% of methane and 60% of anthropogenic nitrous oxide emissions (IPCC, 1996). In the following chapters the mechanisms, factors, estimates of the greenhouse gas emission from soil have been discussed.

ESTIMATES OF GREENHOUSE GAS EMISSION

Initiatives have been taken at international level to estimate the emission of greenhouse gases from various sources (Table 2). The total annual injection of methane into the atmosphere from all sources in the world is estimated to be 535 Tg yr^{-1} (1 Tg = 10^{12} g). India's total contribution to global methane emission from all sources is only 18.5 Tg yr^{-1}. Agriculture, largely rice paddies, and ruminant animal production, is a major (68%) source of this emission. The continuously flooded rice fields emit methane because anoxic conditions favour methanogenesis. The contribution of Indian paddies to this is estimated to be only 3.6 Tg yr^{-1} (Garg and Shukla, 2002). The main reason of low methane emission from rice fields in India is that the soils of major rice growing areas have very low organic carbon and not all paddies are continuously flooded.

Nitrous oxide, which is present in the atmosphere at a very low concentration (310 ppbv), is increasing slowly at the rate of about 0.25% per year. But inspite of its low concentration and slow rise, N_2O assumes greater importance because of its longer life-time (166 years) and greater global warming potential than CO_2 (about 310 times more than that of CO_2). Both fertilized and unfertilized soils emit nitrous oxide. While the fertilizer is the source in case of fertilized soils, the basic nitrogen of the soil contributes to the release of this gas in unfertilized soils. Estimates of total nitrous oxides released from Indian agriculture are low (0.2 Tg yr^{-1}) due to generally low native soil fertility of Indian soils and relatively use of lower amount of fertilizers, as compared to the western world.

The fixation of CO_2 by the agriculture is quite large but its estimates are generally not provided because of continuous consumption of its products by the human beings and other secondary consumers. In India, fixation of CO_2 becomes more important because the country use 190 million-hectare land for farming. The estimated dry biomass production from agriculture in India is almost 800 Tg every year. This is equivalent to fixation of 320 Tg of C or 1000 Tg of CO_2 per annum. Only a part of this is retained over time as the body weight of human beings and other consumers, the rest is released back to atmosphere.

POSSIBLE MEASURES TO MITIGATE GREENHOUSE EFFECT

Alarmed by the possible impact of the global climatic change on the quality of life of human beings; efforts are being made all over the world to develop strategies to mitigate its negative effects, some of these are given in Table 3. There are four major ways agriculture may participate in or be influenced by greenhouse gas mitigation efforts: (a) agriculture may need to reduce emissions because it releases substantial amounts of greenhouse gases, (b) it may enhance its absorption of greenhouse gases by expanding sinks, (c) it may provide products, which substitute for greenhouse gas emission-intensive products displacing emissions and d) it may find itself operating in a world where commodity and input prices have been altered by greenhouse gas emission related policies.

One of the most promising strategies for mitigating methane emission from rice cultivation is altering water management, particularly promoting mid-season aeration by short-term drainage. Improving organic matter management by promoting aerobic degradation through composting or incorporating into soil during off-season drain-period is another promising technique. Organic amendments to flooded soils increase methane production and emission. However, application of well-fermented manure like biogas slurry reduces this emission. In addition, nitrification inhibitors have been shown to inhibit methane emission. Another mitigation option may be the use of different rice cultivars as cultivars grown under similar conditions show pronounced variations in methane emissions. Screening of rice cultivars with few unproductive tillers, small root system, high root oxidative activity and high harvest index are ideal for mitigating methane emission in rice fields. Combined with a package of technologies methane emission can best be reduced by (a) the practice of midseason drainage instead of continuous flooding, (b) direct crop establishment like dry seeded rice, and (c) use of low C: N organic manure and biogas slurry. Appropriate crop management practices, which lead to increase N-use efficiency and yield, hold the key to reduce nitrous oxide emissions. Site-specific nutrient management, fertilizer placement, timing, proper type of fertilizer are some of the practices that supply nutrients in a better accordance with plant demands. Curtailing the nitrification process by the use of nitrification inhibitor may decrease nitrous oxide emission from soil. No-till agriculture that increases C-storage in the soil is one example of a greenhouse gas mitigating practices.

There has been a boost in the agricultural research worldover for understanding the effects of climate change. Nations should come forward together with firm commitments to reduce the emissions of greenhouse gases. Global awareness should be generated about the negative consequences of enhanced greenhouse effect. The governments should form such policies that will help in reducing the emissions of greenhouse gases. Land management systems should be changed so as to reduce methane and nitrous oxide emissions from soil, e.g. intermittent drainage, use of suitable cultivars, and nitrification inhibitors, slow release fertilizers and desired water management practices.

CHAPTER 2

Emission of methane
from soil

H. PATHAK, S. KUMAR, NIVETA JAIN *and* S. MITRA

"Man must go back to nature for information."—Thomas Paine

METHANE IS THE SIMPLEST hydrocarbon having four hydrogen atoms covalently linked to one central carbon atom. Methane molecule has a tetrahedral shape, the four hydrogen atoms occupying the corners of a regular tetrahedron with carbon atom at its center, the formula being CH_4. It is a colourless, odourless gas with melting point $-183°C$ and boiling point $-164°C$ and at room temperature, it is less dense than air. It is sparingly soluble in water (17 mg L^{-1} at 35°C). Methane is combustible and a mixture of about 10% methane in air is explosive. It is not toxic when inhaled, but can produce suffocation by reducing the concentration of inhaled oxygen. Methane is synthesized commercially through the distillation of bituminous coal, or by heating a mixture of carbon and hydrogen. It can be produced in the laboratory by heating sodium acetate with sodium hydroxide or by the reaction of water on aluminum carbide (Al_4C_3).

METHANE AS A NATURAL GAS

Migeotte (1948), who observed strong absorption bands in the infrared region of electromagnetic spectrum caused by atmospheric methane, discovered the presence of methane in the atmosphere. In the early 1970s, Ehhalt and Heidt (1973) measured vertical profiles of methane concentration in the atmosphere of Northern Hemisphere and reported that methane had nearly a uniform distribution in the troposphere with an average concentration of 1.41 ppmV. Ehhalt (1978) subsequently showed a latitudinal gradient of methane concentration with a lower value, about 1.3 ppmV, in Southern Hemisphere than that in the Northern Hemisphere. From these measurements, it was estimated that a total amount of about 4 Pg (1 Pg = 10^{15} g) of methane was present in the atmosphere and the methane cycle contributed 1% to the atmospheric carbon cycle.

Beginning in the decade of 1980s, the evidence for the rapid increase in the concentration of atmospheric methane was reported by time-series measurements of the atmospheric components at many different locations (Blake *et al.*, 1982). The measurements on ice cores at Byrd Station and Dye, both in Antarctica, showed that the concentration of atmospheric methane was around 0.35 ppmV about 20,000 years ago (≈ last glaciation) in comparison to the mean pre-industrial level of about 0.7 ppmV and the current atmospheric concentration of 1.72 ppmV. It has been predicted that by the year 2100 methane levels may reach 3.0 to 4.0 ppmV (US Environmental Protection Agency, 1991). Methane in the atmosphere interacts with infrared radiations contributing to the global warming. The presence of 1.5 ppmV of methane in the atmosphere increases the global average surface temperature by about 1.3 K (Donner and Ramanathan, 1980).

Methane is one of the important greenhouse gases whose concentration in the atmosphere is increasing at the rate of 0.3% yr^{-1} (Prinn, 1995). It accounts for 15-20% of the total enhanced global warming (IPCC, 1996). One of the main anthropogenic sources of methane are the lowland rice fields. Waterlogging in a rice field creates an anoxic environment, which is conducive for methane production by the anaerobic methanogenic bacteria. In order to meet the demand of exploding population, the world's annual rice production needs to be increased by about 65% of the present level over the next three decades, i.e. an increase of 1.7% per annum (IRRI, 1997). In South Asia, the rice production would have to be doubled by the year 2020. Therefore, more intensive rice cultivation is required posing a concern for methane emission from the rice fields. This chapter deals with (i) the processes responsible for methane formation and emission from soil, (ii) factors affecting the emission, (iii) estimates of methane emission from rice fields, and (iv) strategies to reduce the emission.

SOURCES AND SINKS OF ATMOSPHERIC METHANE

The concentration of the atmospheric methane is controlled by the difference in its emission rates from various sources and removal rates mainly through the photochemical reactions in the atmosphere. At present, the emission of CH_4 exceeds its removal, and therefore its concentration is increasing. A wide range of natural and anthropogenic sources of atmospheric CH_4 has been identified and the strength of the emissions from individual sources has been estimated (Table 1). The total annual global emission of methane is estimated to be about 535 Tg (IPCC, 1996), of

Table 1. Global sources and sinks of atmospheric methane

Sources/sinks	Methane emission ($Tg\ yr^{-1}$)	
	Range	Average
Natural		
Wetlands	55-150	115
Termites	10-50	20
Oceans, fresh water	5-50	15
Others	10-40	15
Total	110-210	160
Anthropogenic		
Fossil fuel (coal/gas production/ distribution)	70-120	100
Cattle	65-100	85
Rice paddies	20-100	60
Other sources		
Biomass burning	20-80	40
Landfills	20-70	40
Animal waste	20-30	25
Domestic sewage	15-80	25
Total	300-450	375
Total identified sources	410-660	535
Total sinks	430-600	515
Atmospheric increase	35-40	37

Source: IPCC (1996)

which about 70% is of anthropogenic origin. Fossil fuel burning, cattle, and rice fields are the major sources of anthropogenic methane (Figure 1). However, the strength of an individual source is highly uncertain and wide variations among different estimates are observed due to lack of direct measurements and extreme temporal and spatial variability in methane emissions from different natural and anthropogenic sources.

The major sink for atmospheric methane is its reaction with OH radical in the troposphere, whose concentration is controlled by a complex set of reactions involving CH_4, CO, NOx, and tropospheric O_3. Microbial oxidation of atmospheric methane in soil is the only known biological sink that consumes up to 10% of the total global emission (Adamsen and King, 1993). However, land management, nitrogen fertilizers and soil reactions significantly affect the sink strength.

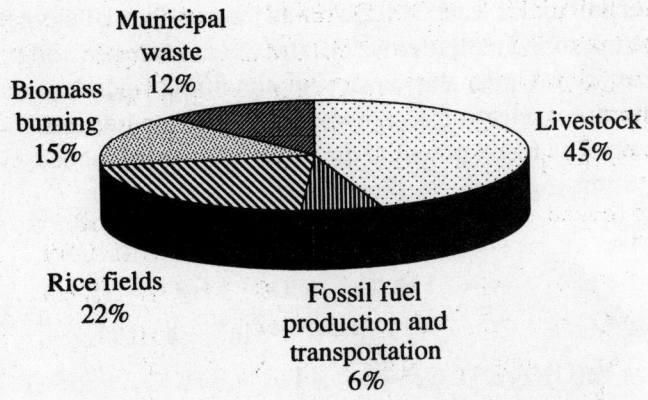

Figure 1: Major contributors of atmospheric methane.

WETLAND RICE FIELDS AS A SOURCE OF METHANE

Paddy fields are important sources of methane emission. Methane emission from rice fields was noted by Harrison and Aiyer as early as 1913, however, the first *in situ* measurement of the methane flux was done in California, USA, in the late 1970s (Cicerone and Shetter, 1981), followed by the extensive studies in several countries of the world (Aulakh *et al.*, 2001). These field experiments stressed the importance of rice plant as a pipe for methane transport from soil to the atmosphere. At present, the methane source strength of wetland rice fields is estimated to be 60 Tg yr^{-1}, with a range of 20–100 Tg yr^{-1} (IPCC, 1996). This estimate is still tentative and efforts are being made to make it more realistic. For this purpose, IPCC has started a worldwide campaign to update the inventory of methane emission from various sources. In India, the Ministry of Environment and Forests is coordinating this campaign.

METHANOGENESIS

The biological formation of methane, termed as methanogenesis, is a geochemically important process that occurs in all anaerobic environments in which organic matter undergoes decomposition. The biogenic methane results from the metabolic activities of a small but highly specific bacterial group that are the terminal members of the food chain in their ecosystem and are called methanogens. Methane is produced by the reduction of soil organic carbon under anaerobic conditions having redox potential less than –150 mV (Wang *et al.*, 1993). Under an oxidized environment, aerobic decomposition of organic carbon occurs with the consequent release of carbon dioxide.

Anaerobic conditions develop in wetland rice fields as a result of submergence of soil under water, which limits the transport of oxygen into the soil and the microbial activities render the water-saturated soil practically devoid of oxygen. Under this anaerobic condition, microorganisms start utilizing alternative electron acceptors for their respiration, causing further soil reduction. The redox potential drops sharply in a sequence, eventually leading to methanogenesis, as shown below:

$$CH_2O + O_2 \longrightarrow CO_2 + H_2O \qquad\qquad -475\,kJ$$

$$5\,CH_2O + 4\,NO_3^- \longrightarrow 4\,HCO_3^- + CO_2 + 3\,H_2O \qquad -448\,kJ$$

$$CH_2O + 2\,MnO_2 + CO_2 + H_2O \longrightarrow 2\,Mn^{++} + 4\,HCO_3^- \qquad -349\,kJ$$

$$CH_2O + 4\,Fe(OH)_3 + 7\,CO_2 \longrightarrow 4\,Fe^{++} + 8\,HCO_3^- + 3\,H_2O \quad -114\,kJ$$

$$2\,CH_2O + SO_4^- \longrightarrow H_2S + 2\,HCO_3^- \qquad\qquad -77\,kJ$$

$$2\,CH_2O + H_2O \longrightarrow CH_4 + CO_2 + H_2O \qquad\qquad -58\,kJ$$

The sequence is strictly in accordance with the yield of free energy. The process of soil reduction tends to stabilize the soil pH to near neutral, which is optimal for methanogenesis (Oremland, 1988). High salinity and sulphate concentration increase the competitive interactions of sulphur-reducing bacteria and methanogens. Application of organic manure and fertilizers, and submergence under deep water increase the population and activities of methanogenic bacteria in paddy soils.

Under anaerobic and reduced conditions, methanogens produce methane either through the reduction of carbon dioxide by hydrogen, known as 'hydrogenotrophic pathway' or the fermentation of acetate to methane and carbon dioxide, called 'aceticlastic pathway'. In nature, the later mechanism accounts for about two-thirds of the methane emission from soil. These bacteria being strictly anaerobic, convert the fermentation products, notably CO_2, H_2, esters and salts of methanoic acid (HCOOH) formed by other microorganisms, into CH_4. The reactions with reference to the type of methanogens involved in forming CH_4 as an end product are given below:

(a) Reduction of CO_2 by H_2 through chemoautotrophic methanogens:

$$CO_2 + 4\,H_2 \longrightarrow CH_4 + 2\,H_2O$$

(b) Several strains of methanogens also use HCOOH or CO as a substrate for producing CH_4 in addition to CO_2 and H_2:

$$4\,HCOOH \longrightarrow CH_4 + 3\,CO_2 + 2\,H_2O$$

$$4\,CO + 2\,H_2O \longrightarrow CH_4 + 3\,CO_2$$

(c) Methane is also produced by methylotrophic methanogens, which use methyl-group containing substrates such as methanol, acetate and trimethylamine:

$$4 \, CH_3OH \longrightarrow 3 \, CH_4 + CO_2 + 2 \, H_2O$$

$$CH_3COOH \longrightarrow CH_4 + CO_2$$

$$4 \, (CH_3)_3N + 6 \, H_2O \longrightarrow 9 \, CH_4 + 3 \, CO_2 + 4 \, NH_3$$

METHANE CONSUMPTION

There are some aerobic ecosystems which function as sinks for methane. Such a transformation of CH_4 to CO_2 by the oxidation process is carried out by methanotropic bacteria. About 80% of the potential diffusive CH_4 flux through the soil-water interface is oxidized in the oxic surface layers, indicating that CH_4 oxidising bacteria in the shallow oxic surface layers of rice fields operate very efficiently. The oxidation pathway is represented in Scheme 1.

$$CH_4 \xrightarrow{\text{Monoxygenase}} CH_3CHO \xrightarrow[\text{dehydrogenase}]{\text{Methanol}} HCHO \xrightarrow[\text{dehydrogenase}]{\text{Formaldehyde}} HCOOH \xrightarrow[\text{dehydrogenase}]{\text{Formate}} CO_2$$

Scheme 1. The oxidation pathway of methane

Methanotrophs are a subset of physiological group of methylotrophs, which utilize a variety of one-carbon compounds. Some of the microorganisms responsible for the oxidation of methane are strictly aerobic, obligate methylo- or methano-trophic eubacteria. These microorganisms can use methane and other C_1-compounds such as methanol as substrates. Ammonium could possibly inhibit the oxidation of methane by constraining the availability of oxygen while sulphate may cause a significant removal of methane from soil.

$$CH_4 + SO_4^{2-} \longrightarrow HCO_3^- + HS^- + H_2O$$

ESTIMATES OF METHANE EMISSION

The estimates of methane emission from rice fields have varied considerably over time with the advances in the method of measurement and availability of more and more data. The best estimate of the global emission of methane from rice fields is in the range of 30-70 Tg yr^{-1} (Neue, 1997), based on various model calculations by different groups. Methane emissions from different countries are given in Table 2. The measurements in rice paddies at various locations have shown that there are large temporal variations of methane emissions differing markedly with climate, soil and paddy characteristics, fertilizers applied, organic matter content and other

Table 2. Seasonal methane emission from rice fields in different countries

Country	Average $(kg\ ha^{-1})$
Philippines	175
Vietnam	336
China	256
Indonesia	161
Thailand	49
Korea	367
Japan	182
India	45

Source: Gupta and Mitra (1999)

agricultural practices. Moreover, rice is grown in different ecosystems, i.e. irrigated, rainfed and deep-water contributing 75, 22 and 3% of the total CH_4 emission from rice fields, respectively (Neue, 1997). Most of the methane emitted from rice fields is regarded to be from the Asia as it has 90% of the total world rice harvested area, out of which about 52% is in China and India (IRRI, 1995). The estimates of methane emissions from Indian paddy fields are of special significance as India has 42.2 million ha of land under rice cultivation, of which 16.4 million ha is irrigated and the remaining is rainfed (19.7 and 5.9 million ha lowland and upland, respectively). Methane emission from rice paddies in India is $3.64 \pm 1.26\ Mt\ yr^{-1}$ (Table 3).

PROCESSES REGULATING THE TRANSFER OF METHANE FROM SOIL TO THE ATMOSPHERE

The three processes that regulate the transfer of methane from soil to the atmosphere are: (i) vascular transport, (ii) ebullition, and (iii) diffusion.

Vascular transport

Methane is emitted from paddy fields mostly by transport through rice plants, which act as bundles of chimneys for transporting methane from the rhizosphere to the atmosphere (Figure 2). Aerenchyma tissues, in a number of aquatic plants as well as in rice, helps in the transport of oxygen and some other gases. The path of methane through a rice plant includes diffusion into the root, movement through cortex and aerenchyma and release to the atmosphere through micropores in the leaf sheath. Methane transport capacity of a rice plant is dependent mainly on its size. The con-

Table 3. Methane budget estimates from Indian rice fields

Water regime		Harvested area (Mha)	Emission (g m^{-2})	Seasonal integrated flux (g m^{-2})	Total emission (Tg yr^{-1})
Upland		6.35			
Lowland	Rainfed Flood-prone	4.23	16 (10-20)	19 ± 6.0	0.8 ± 0.25
	Drought-prone	6.77	8 (0-10)	7.3 ± 2.3	0.49 ± 0.16
	Irrigated Continuously-flooded	6.77	20	15.6 ± 6.3	1.06 ± 0.43
	Intermittently-flooded Single aeration	9.92	10 (4-14)	7.3 ± 2.3	0.72 ± 0.23
	Multiple aeration	5.74	4 (2-6)	1.58 ± 0.74	0.091 ± 0.04
	Deepwater Water depth 50-100 cm	2.54	16 (12-20)	19.0 ± 6.0	0.48 ± 0.15
Total					3.64 ± 1.26

Source: Gupta and Mitra (1999)

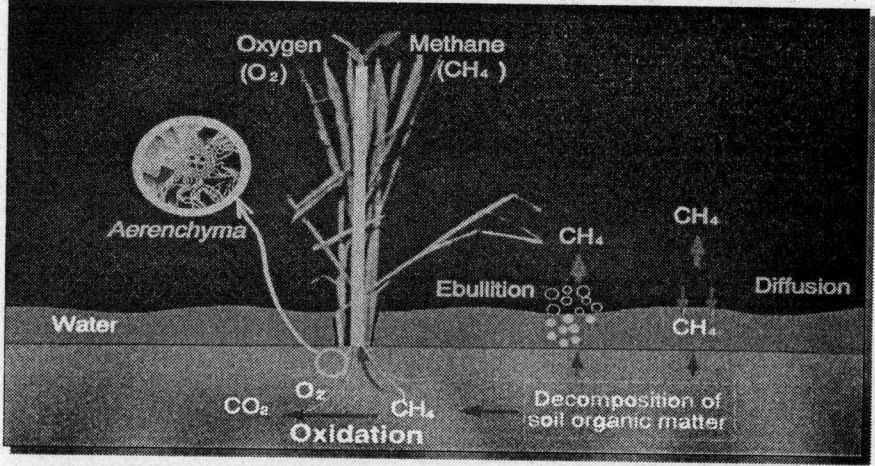

Figure 2: Scheme of methane production and emission in a rice field.
(*Courtesy:* H.U. Neue, IRRI)

cept of plant-mediated transport as the predominant mechanism for the emission of methane from the rice fields has been established by comparative measurements in rice-planted and un-planted soils. It has been observed that with the growth of rice plants, there is an increase in the contribution of plant-mediated methane emission. Some researchers have suggested a slightly different pathway (Wang *et al.*, 1997). According to them, about 50% of the methane is released from the leaf blades before shoot elongation, whereas only a small amount is emitted through leaves as plants grow older. In addition to the presence of micropores on leaf sheath, cracks in junction points of internodes have also been observed. Although methane can also be released through panicles but this pathway is followed negligibly as long as leaves and nodes are not submerged. Methane emission rates increased linearly with the number of nodal culms, indicating a direct proportionality between the number of culms and the release sites.

Ebullition

Many researchers have identified ebullition of gases entrapped in sediments and peats as a possible form of methane release to the atmosphere. The ebullition process could be influenced by factors like wind speed, temperature, solar radiation, water level, depth of water table and atmospheric pressure. It has been observed that unplanted fields emit 50% of the amount of methane emitted by the fields planted with rice. The methane ebullition is important during the early stage of flooding, when rice plants are small, whereas vascular transport becomes more important as the rice plants grow older.

Diffusion

Diffusion of gases in water is 10^4-times slower than in air, and therefore, exchange of gases almost stops when soils are waterlogged. The actual diffusion of methane from rice fields is a function of its supply to the floodwater, its concentration in the floodwater and prevailing wind speed. Diffusion through the floodwater is usually less than 1% of the total flux. However, the rate-limiting step in plant-mediated CH_4 transport (vascular transport) is its diffusion across the root/shoot junction.

TEMPORAL AND SPATIAL VARIATION IN METHANE EMISSION

The methane emission generally shows strong diurnal and seasonal variations. The seasonal variations in methane emission depend on factors like growing stage of rice, temperature, day-length, solar radiation, humidity, water regimes, fertilization, weeding, etc. During the early vegetative period, maximum methane emission occurs at both noon and night, while during the late vegetative period, it occurs only at night. It is due to transportation of less oxygen to the root system of rice plants at night resulting in less methane oxidation and higher emission. The temporal and spatial variations of methane production are related to rice root biomass, which might depend on cultivars and soil.

FACTORS REGULATING METHANE EMISSION

Methane production and consumption in soil are the biologically-mediated processes, and therefore, are affected by the prevalent weather conditions, water regime, soil properties and various cultural practices like irrigation and drainage, organic amendments, fertilization and rice cultivars. We shall discuss these factors individually.

Temperature

Temperature plays an important role in the activity of soil microorganisms, including those involved in methane emission. The temperature influences methane production by regulating (i) anaerobic carbon mineralization and availability of alternative electron acceptors, and (ii) methanogenic activity. At a higher temperature mineralization increases and more carbon substrate becomes available, resulting in a faster depletion of the alternative electron acceptor pool. However, the influence of temperature on methane production is mainly through its effect on methanogenic activity. Most of the methanogenic bacteria display optimum rates of methane production at around 30-35°C with very little methanogenesis between 5 and 15°C (Yagi *et al.*, 1997). The methane emission rate increases sharply when the soil temperature rises from 10 to 35°C, corresponding with a temperature coefficient (Q_{10}) of about 4 (Holzapfel-Pschorn and Seiler, 1986).

pH

Most of the methanogens are neutrophilic, hence methane production is most efficient in the pH range 6.4–7.8. Methanogenesis is a highly pH-sensitive process and a small change in the pH value sharply lowers the methane production. Below pH 5.8 and above 8.8, methane production in the soil suspension is almost completely inhibited.

Redox potential (Eh)

Methanogenesis occurs only under anaerobic conditions. A sufficiently low value (–150 mV) of redox potential (*Eh*) is required for methane production and it is negatively related to methane emission. In soils with high contents of Fe and organic matter, the *Eh* value falls to –50 mV and may slowly decline further to -200 mV over a period of one month. Soils low in active-Fe with high organic matter attain lower *Eh* values much faster, may be within a week after submergence. Flooded rice soils may have *Eh* values as low as –250 to –300 mV, while *Eh* of –150 to –190 mV is needed for methane formation (Wang *et al.*, 1993). However, there are reports that CH_4 production in freshly flooded rice soils is initiated much earlier than generally expected in spite of high *Eh* values. This early initiation of methane production is due to the presence of enough viable methanogenic archaea in the soils (Roy *et al.*, 1997).

Organic amendments

Application of organic manure and crop residues enhances the methanogenesis process. The amount of methane formed in paddy soils is positively correlated with soil organic-carbon and water-soluble organic-carbon provided other factors, such as bacterial population and oxidizing capacity of the soil are not limiting. Incorporation of rice straw in the soil increases methane production by 120–800% over that of unammended soil. Even the method of incorporation of straw is also important in regulating methane emission. Methane emission is highest with the incorporation of straw followed by straw compost, zero tillage with straw mulching and least with straw ash application (Chaareonsi *et al.*, 2000). Application of biogas spent slurry as a manure results in lowering of methane emission compared to application of farmyard manure (FYM) from rice·fields (Debnath *et al.*, 1996). Use of biogas slurry, therefore, could be a practical mitigation option for minimizing methane flux from flooded rice fields.

It has been found that growing of azolla for biological nitrogen fixation could enhance methane emission from rice fields due to mediation of methane transport from floodwater of rice soil into the atmosphere (Ying *et al.*, 2000). The presence of azolla could modify the chemical properties of soil, stimulating methane production and decreasing the *in situ* methane removal. It also lowers the *Eh* value, which increases the methane production. Also, NH_4^+-N content gets lowered, leading to reduction in biological methane oxidation and porosity of rice soil, resulting in higher emission of methane.

Cultivars

Plant influences the methane efflux by (i) providing channels (aerenchyma) for the transport of methane from soil to the atmosphere, (ii) releasing root exudates or root autolysis products to methanogenic bacteria, and (iii) creating oxic environment in the anoxic soil through the transport of O_2 into the rhizosphere stimulating the oxidation of methane and inhibiting methanogenesis (Wassmann *et al.*, 2000). There are significant variations in the quantities of methane emitted from soils growing different cultivars. Early-maturing cultivars emit less methane compared to that from late-maturing cultivars. The high yielding varieties like IR-64 show moderately high emissions (Setyanto *et al.*, 2000). Such differences in CH_4 emission from the rice cultivars could be due to the differences in amounts of root exudates produced per plant, the CH_4 oxidizing capacity of the roots, and the population level of methanogenic bacteria in roots.

Mineral fertilizers

Methane fluxes are strongly influenced by the type, method and the rate of fertilizer application. Sulphate-containing fertilizers reduce methane emission. It has been observed that methane emission, on an average, decreased by 42 and 60% in the ammonium sulphate treatments and 7 and 14% in the urea treatments at rates of 100 and 300 kg N ha^{-1}, respectively, compared to control (Cai *et al.*, 1997). Phosphogypsum, a sulphate-containing by-product of industrial production of phosphoric acid, reduces methane emission by 56-73% when applied in combination with urea. In a field study P applied as single super phosphate (SSP) inhibit methane emission from a flooded field plot planted under rice (Adhya *et al.*, 1998). Supplementary addition of K_2SO_4 with K_2HPO_4, mimicked the inhibitory effect of SSP on methane production. In practice, the use of SSP in rice cultivation could mitigate methane production, in addition to supplying P to the crops.

Water management

The water regime of soil is an important factor for the gas exchange between soil and atmosphere and has a direct impact on the processes involved in methane emission. For methanogenesis to take place, it is of primary importance that the soils should have enough moisture to create an anoxic condition. Drainage is a major modifier of seasonal methane emission pattern. A single mid-season drainage may reduce seasonal methane emission. This emission could be reduced further by intermittent irrigation yielding a 30% reduction as compared to mid-season drainage (Lu *et al.*, 2000). Thus, intermittent flooding practice is very efficient in reducing methane emission without a significant effect on grain yield. The percolating water also transports organic solutes and dissolved gases into the subsoil or groundwater where leached methane may be oxidized or released to the atmosphere. In a four-year study in northern India, it has been observed that low emissions are indirectly caused by high percolation rates of the soil and the frequent water replenishments cause constant inflow of oxygen in the soil (Jain *et al.*, 2000).

Salts

Methane emission is inversely related to salinity and sulphate concentration in soil. The sulphates and sulphides may be toxic to methanogens and hence reduce methane production. Between the two main pathways of methane formation, the reduction of CO_2 is less susceptible to salt (NaCl) than the decomposition of acetic acid (Saenjan and Wada, 1990).

Soil texture

Soil texture and mineralogy, through their effect on puddling, can affect percolation rate of water and thereby net emission of methane in waterlogged paddy soils. Clay soils form cracks on drying and thus facilitate the release of entrapped methane into the atmosphere.

MITIGATION STRATEGY FOR METHANE EMISSION

The possible strategies for mitigating methane emission from rice cultivation can be made by controlling production, oxidation and transport of methane from soil to the atmosphere.

- Methane emission varies markedly with water regimes. Altering water management, particularly promoting mid-season aeration by short-term drainage is one of the most promising strategies for reducing methane emission.

- Improving organic matter management by promoting aerobic degradation through composting or incorporating it into soil during off-season drained period is another promising technique.
- A frequently suggested mitigation option is the use of sulphate-containing fertilizers such as ammonium sulphate because the sulphate-reducing bacteria can out-compete methane producing bacteria and thus reduce the amount of methane produced from a rice field.
- In addition to their role in controlling various processes of N losses, nitrification inhibitors like nitrapyrin have been shown to inhibit methane emission from flooded soil planted to rice.
- Organic amendments to flooded soils increase methane production and emission. However, application of fermented manure like biogas slurry reduces this emission.
- Another mitigation option may be the use of different rice cultivars as cultivars grown under similar conditions show pronounced variations in methane emission. Screening of rice cultivars with few unproductive tillers, small root system, high root oxidative activity and high harvest index are ideal for mitigating methane emission in rice fields.

The Intergovernmental Panel on Climate Change (IPCC) has recommended immediate reductions of 15-20% in anthropogenic emission of methane to stabilize its atmospheric concentration at the 1990-level (IPCC, 1996). Manipulation of all or some of the factors causing variability in CH_4 emission rates mentioned above might offer a way in which this target could be met. Moreover, the strategies to reduce the methane emission should not have any adverse effect on crop yields. Environment-friendly technologies must consider both for maintaining, and even increasing soil fertility, and mitigating methane emissions. The only feasible way in which these two opposing requirements may be met is to follow crop management practices that reduce methane emissions without affecting the crop yield. Combined with a package of technologies, the methane emission can best be reduced by: (a) following the practice of midseason drainage instead of continuous flooding, (b) using sulphate-containing fertilizers, (c) direct crop establishment like dry-seeded rice, and (d) using low C: N organic manure.

There are many microbial, climatic, hydrological, soil, crop and management factors that control the production, consumption and transport of methane in rice ecosystem in different ways. However, the extent of their effect on the production and emission of methane has not been evaluated quantitatively. The precise estimates are difficult also due to the large spatial and temporal variabilities in methane emission and its measurement at different sites due to variations in climate, soil properties, duration and pattern of flooding, rice cultivars and crop growth, organic amendments, and fertilization and cultural practices. Therefore, attention must focus on developing simple and accurate technologies in quantifying methane emissions for different land use types and developing process-based models to obtain reliable estimates of methane emission at regional and global levels. The efficacy of various mitigation technologies needs to be tested in farmers' fields. Moreover, these technologies need to be assessed for non-target effects and economic feasibility.

CHAPTER 3

Nitrous oxide emission from soil

H. PATHAK, ARTI BHATIA, S. PRASAD *and* V. SHARMA

"Whether man is disposed to yield to nature or to oppose her, he can not do without a correct understanding of her language."—Jean Rostand

NITROUS OXIDE (N_2O) is an important greenhouse gas. With its current concentration of 310 ppbV, it accounts for approximately 5% of the total greenhouse effect. It is also responsible for the destruction of the stratospheric ozone. The concern for the presence of nitrous oxide in atmosphere becomes larger due to the fact that it has a lifetime of 166 ± 16 years in the atmosphere. Soil is considered to be one of the major sources of nitrous oxide emission, contributing 65% to the total global emission. Annual emission of N_2O-N from agricultural system amounts to 6.3 Tg which includes the direct emission from agricultural soil and animal system and the indirect emission from agricultural soil through loss of nitrogen to aquatic system and atmosphere. From agricultural perspective, nitrous oxide emission from soil represents a loss of soil nitrogen, reducing the nitrogen (N)-use efficiency. The soil receiving chemical-fertilizer nitrogen and biologically-fixed nitrogen contributes to nitrous oxide emission during the processes of denitrification and nitrification. Due to advent of modern agriculture, consumption of nitrogenous fertilizer has risen sharply all over the world. This is expected to increase further to meet the food demand of growing population. Consequently, the emission of nitrous oxide from soil would also increase. Any attempt to reduce this emission has a great significance as it will not only reduce the atmospheric pollution but also increase fertilizer-use efficiency. The pre-requisite of developing management practices to minimize nitrous oxide emission from managed ecosystems is the understanding of the sources and factors controlling its emission. This chapter deals with the (i) processes responsible for nitrous oxide formation and emission from soil, (ii) factors affecting this emission, (iii) estimates of nitrous oxide emission from agriculture, and (iv) strategies to reduce nitrous oxide emission from soil.

NITROUS OXIDE AS A NATURAL GAS

Nitrous oxide was first discovered and prepared in 1793 by an English scientist and clergyman, Joseph Priestley. Nitrous oxide, also known as laughing gas, a term coined by Humphrey Davy of the Pneumatic Institute, Bristol, England, is a colourless, almost odourless gas with molecular weight 44, specific gravity 1.53, and boiling point $-89°C$. The atmospheric abundance, life-time, sources, and sinks of nitrous oxide are given in Table 1 in Chapter 1. The concentration of N_2O in the atmosphere before the industrial revolution was 280-290 ppbV. It has increased by about 8% since then and is currently increasing at 0.22 ± 0.02 % yr^{-1}. This increase can be mainly attributed to anthropogenic activities.

MECHANISM OF NITROUS OXIDE FORMATION IN SOIL

The emission of nitrous oxide is an integral part of the N-transformation processes in soil (Figure 1). The biological processes of denitrification, ni-

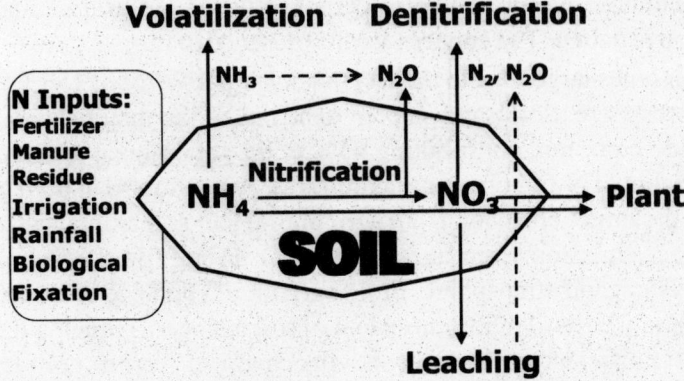

Figure 1: Nitrogen in soil-plant-atmosphere systems.

trification, dissimilatory nitrate reduction and assimilatory nitrate reduction, as well as the abiological reactions of chemodenitrification are the possible mechanisms of nitrous oxide emission from soil. However, it has been established that denitrification and nitrification are the most important mechanisms others contributing very little (<1%) to this pool.

Nitrification contributes to nitrous oxide emission through the biological oxidation of ammonium (NH_4^+-N) to nitrate (NO_3^--N) following ammonium fertilizer or ammonia forming fertilizer addition in aerobic soil. The scheme of reactions in the nitrification process is shown in Figure 2.

Nitrification

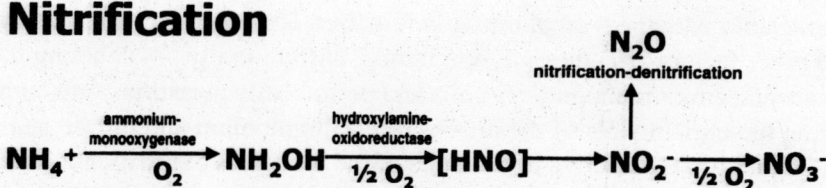

$$N_2O$$
nitrification-denitrification

$$NH_4^+ \xrightarrow[\text{O}_2]{\text{ammonium-monooxygenase}} NH_2OH \xrightarrow[\text{½ O}_2]{\text{hydroxylamine-oxidoreductase}} [HNO] \longrightarrow NO_2^- \xrightarrow{\text{½ O}_2} NO_3^-$$

Denitrification

$$NO$$

$$NO_3 \xrightarrow[\text{reductase}]{\text{nitrate}} NO_2 \xrightarrow[\text{reductase}]{\text{nitrite}} [NO] \xrightarrow[\text{reductase}]{\text{nitric oxide}} N_2O \xrightarrow[\text{reductase}]{\text{nitrous oxide}} N_2$$

Figure 2: Emission of nitric oxide by nitrification and denitrification processes.

A simple scheme of denitrification is shown in Figure 2. Denitrification occurs when nitrate is present in anaerobic soil developed wherever the microbial demand for oxygen exceeds the diffusion-mediated supply. This may well occur where oxygen diffusion is impeded by water, either at the centers of soil or in water saturated regions or wherever the local oxygen demand is exceptionally high. Denitrification in soils also consumes nitrous oxide through the reduction of nitrous oxide to nitrogen. This has been illustrated in the hole and pipe model (Figure 3). Hence denitrification may serve either as a source or as a sink for nitrous oxide.

The relative contribution of nitrification and denitrification processes in nitrous oxide emission from soil is difficult to assess and is likely to vary

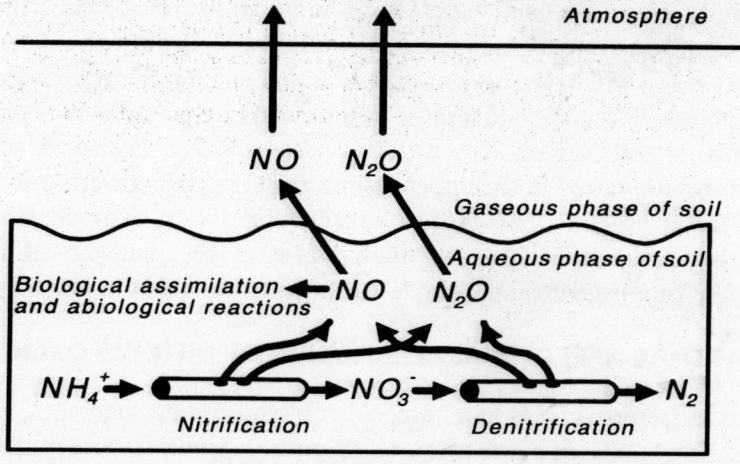

Figure 3: Hole in the pipe model for emission of nitrous oxide
(Firestone and Davidson, 1989)

appreciably with the type of nitrogen fertilizer, land management, climate and other factors affecting soil conditions. Differentially ^{15}N-labeling the nitrate and ammonium pools in soils and periodically measuring and comparing the enrichments of the nitrous oxide, ammonium and nitrate pools could quantify the relative importance of the processes of nitrification and denitrification in nitrous oxide emission.

OTHER MICROBIAL PROCESSES

Nitrous oxide is also produced by various microorganisms during the following processes:

(i) dissimilatory nitrate reduction,
(ii) respiratory nitrate reduction and
(iii) assimilatory nitrate reduction.

All these metabolic pathways typically produce nitrous oxide but they do not gain energy by producing nitrous oxide. They have thus been named as 'non-respiratory N_2O producers' in contrast to respiratory nitrous oxide producing denitrifiers.

CHEMICAL FORMATION OF NITROUS OXIDE

Nitrous oxide can also be formed by chemical reactions such as decomposition of nitrite or hydroxylamine in acid soils:

$$NH_2OH + HNO_2 \longrightarrow N_2O + 2\,H_2O$$

However, the formation of nitrous oxide by chemical reaction of nitrite and hydroxylamine does not seem to be important since the reaction becomes significant only in the presence of relatively high nitrite concentrations (>1 mM), which are not commonly found in natural environments.

It is generally assumed that most of nitrous oxide production occurs in proximity of soil surface. The nitrous oxide produced deeper in soil is likely to be consumed in the upper soil layer during the upward transport by a diffusive process. This process of reduction of nitrous oxide to nitrogen during diffusion is enhanced when the soil is wet, since the diffusion coefficient of nitrous oxide is much less in water than that in air.

FACTORS AFFECTING THE EMISSION OF NITROUS OXIDE

A range of factors such as moisture, soil, climate and management, affect the emission of nitrous oxide from soil (Figure 4). Some of these important factors are discussed below.

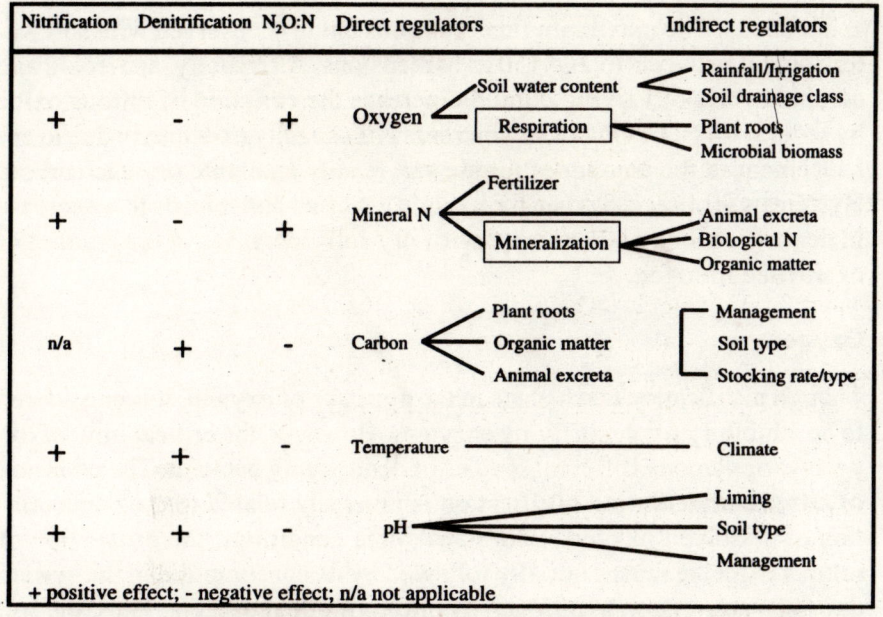

Nitrification	Denitrification	N₂O:N	Direct regulators	Indirect regulators
+	-	+	Oxygen	Soil water content / Respiration — Rainfall/Irrigation, Soil drainage class, Plant roots, Microbial biomass
+	-	+	Mineral N	Fertilizer / Mineralization — Animal excreta, Biological N, Organic matter
n/a	+	-	Carbon	Plant roots, Organic matter, Animal excreta — Management, Soil type, Stocking rate/type
+	+	-	Temperature	Climate
+	+	-	pH	Liming, Soil type, Management

+ positive effect; - negative effect; n/a not applicable

Figure 4: Factors affecting nitrous oxide emission.

Moisture regime

Moisture plays a major role in the emission of nitrous oxide from soil by influencing the nitrification and denitrification processes. Soil water affect directly or indirectly the denitrification through (i) providing suitable conditions for microbial growth and activity, (ii) restricting the supply of oxygen to micro-sites by filling soil pores, (iii) releasing the available carbon and nitrogen substrates through wetting and drying cycles, and (iv) providing a diffusion medium through which substrates and products are moved to and away from soil microorganisms. However, the primary effect of water on nitrous oxide production in aerobic and partially aerobic soils is to restrict soil oxygen levels by reducing the air-water interfacial area within air-filled pores, thus producing the anaerobic condition. Low emission occurs when gravimetric soil water content is less than 30%. Nitrous oxide emission in soil increases with increase in soil moisture content. Generally, an increase in denitrification rates is commonly observed following irrigation and precipitation. When water content is greater than the field capacity, nitrous oxide gets reduced to nitrogen, thereby reducing nitrous oxide fluxes. Due to this reason, lowland rice is not considered to be an important source of atmospheric nitrous oxide. However, in irrigated rice grown in upland conditions, where natural drainage of standing water during crop growth makes the soil sometimes aerobic, emission of nitrous oxide is promoted through enhancement of the nitrification process (Pathak *et al.,* 2002). The maximum flux of nitrous oxide is observed with soil water content between 75 and 150 m bar tensions. Alternately, anaerobic and aerobic cycles of varying duration increase the emission of nitrous oxide by several folds. Drying of soil increases its capacity to denitrify due to enhancement in the amount of nitrate and readily available organic carbon. Hysteresis is observed when moist soils get dried and it leads to a decrease in denitrification, whereas wetting of dry soils increases in the amount of denitrified nitrogen.

Oxygen

Though nitrification takes place in the presence of oxygen, it is considered to be inhibitory for denitrifying enzymes. However, the critical limit of oxygen varies among different species of denitrifying bacteria. The emission of nitrous oxide during nitrification is inversely related to the concentration of dissolved oxygen. Under anaerobic conditions, the production of nitrous oxide increases initially followed by its consumption in the system due to its conversion to nitrogen by nitrous oxide reductase. Thus, the soil can act as a sink for nitrous oxide under anoxic conditions. Nitrous oxide emission is higher in soils with fluctuating redox potential generated by alternate wetting and drying cycles.

pH

Soil acidity, through various mechanisms, may modulate the emission of nitrous oxide, these are:

- The increased soil acidity may lower the decomposition rate of soil organic matter, which reduces the availability of nitrogen substrate for nitrous oxide production.
- A higher soil acidity directly reduces the microbial activity.
- The acidification may severely inhibit nitrous oxide reductase with the result that denitrification will yield more of nitrous oxide than nitrogen.
- The decreasing pH reduces the availability of molybdenum which, in turn, may reduce the synthesis of nitrate reductase which is a molybdo-protein enzyme.
- With decreasing pH, nitrite formed by nitrate reduction cannot undergo further reduction and thus an accumulation of nitrite occurs and leads to the solubilization of aluminum or manganese which might cause toxicity.
- A severe acidification may induce chemical production of nitrous oxide from nitrite.

The optimum pH for nitrous oxide emission via nitrification and denitrification varies with species and age of organisms and the ammonium and nitrate concentrations in soil. Most nitrifying and denitrifying bacteria have optimum pH for growth between 6 and 8. Although denitrification process is favoured at slightly alkaline pH, it can proceed at pH as low as 3.5 and can account for significant nitrogen losses in acid soils.

Soil texture

The effect of soil texture on nitrous oxide emission is probably due to the physical variations in the proportions of air and water. The rates of water infiltration and gas diffusion are highly influenced by soil texture and hence nitrous oxide emission. Higher rates of nitrous oxide emission are obtained in finer-textured soils. Small N additions do not result in an immediate increase in nitrous oxide emission from sandy loam soil but significantly increase nitrous oxide flux from clay loam soil (Mosier *et al.*, 1998). Conversely, highest flux is observed from sandy soil followed by loamy and clayey soil.

Temperature

Nitrous oxide emission increases with rise in soil temperature from 10 to 40°C. However, emission due to denitrification occurs at a very high rate in the temperature range 60-70°C due to a combination of biological and chemical reactions. As the thermophilic temperature approaches, the activities of thermophilic nitrate respirers are enhanced and chemodenitrification reactions dominate. The thawing of frozen soil can lead to a temporal increase in nitrous oxide production. There are reports of brief but vigorous nitrous oxide fluxes during rapid thaw events in spring from sandy loam soil. The production of nitrous oxide is two orders of magnitude higher at thaw in spring than at any time during the rest of the year. This may be due to changes in solubility, production near the soil surface and diffusion of nitrous oxide from lower soil depth.

Fertilizer application

The production of nitrous oxide in soil increases in N-fertilized soils. The form of added N also plays an important role in regulating nitrous oxide emission. The amount of nitrous oxide evolved from plots treated with ammonium sulphate [$(NH_4)_2SO_4$] or urea (NH_2CONH_2) is significantly more than from those plots which receive the same amount of nitrogen as calcium nitrate [$Ca(NO_3)_2$]. It has also been observed that the nitrous oxide emission is larger from soils fertilized with anhydrous ammonia than from those fertilized with nitrate and ammonium salts. This can be attributed to the fact that the customary method of applying anhydrous ammonia by injection into the soil produces highly alkaline zones and results in high nitrous oxide emissions. Studies at the Indian Agricultural Research Institute have shown that urea, which is widely used as a nitrogenous fertilizer in the country, contributes maximum to the nitrous oxide emission. It is followed by ammonium sulphate, ammonium chloride and potassium nitrate from alluvial soil at submerged and field capacity moisture regimes (Majumdar *et al.,* 2000). Data from 104 field experiments all over the world have shown that 2.7% of anhydrous ammonia, 0.44% of ammonium nitrate, 0.25% of ammonium type, 0.11% of urea and 0.05% of nitrate are lost as nitrous oxide (Eichner, 1990). However, this estimate differs significantly from that of Galbally (1985), who reported that 0.5 % of anhydrous ammonia, 0.1% of ammonium nitrate, 0.1% of ammonium type, 0.5% of urea and 0.05% of nitrate are emitted as nitrous oxide. Intergovernmental Panel on Climate Change (IPCC) currently assumes a nitrous oxide emission factor of 1.25% of the fertilizer nitrogen applied. Nitrous oxide emission not only depends on the type of fertilizer nitrogen but also on the mode of its application. The application of urea in plough layers gives less emission of nitrous oxide than band application of urea fertilizer. The emission of different amounts of nitrous oxide from different forms of fertilizer nitrogen suggests that this factor could be an efficient way of limiting the emission. Addition of phosphorus and liming materials can also affect nitrous oxide evolution from soil. However, phosphorus induced emissions are higher than those obtained with calcium carbonate.

Organic manure amendment

Organic amendments such as plant residues, green manure and farmyard manure increase the rates of nitrous oxide emission as niritifiers and denitrifiers use organic carbon compounds as electron donors for energy and synthesis of cellular constituents. Nitrous oxide emission is directly related with biochemical oxygen demand (BOD) of organic amendment applied to the soil. During the first few days after the application of a manure, high emission of nitrous oxide is observed. This emission originates from rapid nitrification and denitrification induced by the manure, since these contain considerable amounts of ammonium and readily-available organic carbon. The worldwide application of manure nitrogen (74.9 Tg yr^{-1}) is in the same range as nitrogen applied as synthetic fertilizer (77.4 Tg yr^{-1}) and therefore, could contribute substantially towards emission of nitrous oxide.

Plant

Apart from its role in providing a channel for transportation of nitrous oxide from soil to the atmosphere, a plant affects the formation of nitrous oxide by influencing the nitrate and carbon contents and the partial pressure of oxygen in soil. Plants can directly influence the availability of nitrate through uptake and assimilation, making it unavailable to denitrification. An indirect effect of nitrate levels arises from the supply of organic matter of root origin. Mineralization and nitrification of this material can potentially provide more nitrates for denitrification and conversely immobilization can reduce nitrate levels. Moreover, nitrous oxide dissolved in water is taken up by the plant roots and transported to the leaves through the transpiration stream. Another indirect effect is the ability of few plants, e.g. rice to supply oxygen at the rhizosphere, which can enhance nitrate content by promoting nitrification. Plant species might differ in their effect on denitrification. Higher rates of denitrification are obtained in soils grown with a legume rather than with a monocotyledonous plant. Crop-specific field management and nitrogen fertilization have great roles in the emission of nitrous oxide, which is due to crop-specific differences in soil nitrate and soil moisture content.

INTERACTIONS OF VARIOUS FACTORS AFFECTING NITROUS OXIDE EMISSION

Organic carbon, oxygen and nitrate content of soils are three important factors that exert a direct effect on nitrous oxide emission. The effects of these primary factors are influenced by a number of secondary interactions. Soil water-content exerts diffusional constraints on soil oxygen. It also influences the availability of organic carbon through wetting and drying cycles. Organic carbon affects nitrate availability, which is manifested through mineralization/immobilization reactions. Nitrate availability is also subjected to diffusional constraints imposed by soil-water content. Soil texture and structure can also influence nitrous oxide emission. Finally, microbial respiration of the available organic carbon can have a dramatic effect on oxygen levels at the micro site level. Thus, heterogeneous nature of the soil matrix makes the relationships more complex and difficult to quantify. Very little information is available on the effect of various factors and their interaction on emission of nitrous oxide. There is a need to make these studies so as to quantify the estimates of nitrous oxide.

PROCESSES REGULATING TRANSFER OF NITROUS OXIDE FROM SOIL TO THE ATMOSPHERE

Vascular transport, ebullition and diffusion are the main pathways by which nitrous oxide formed inside the soil is emitted to the atmosphere (Figure 5). In vascular transport, plants act as bundles of chimneys to

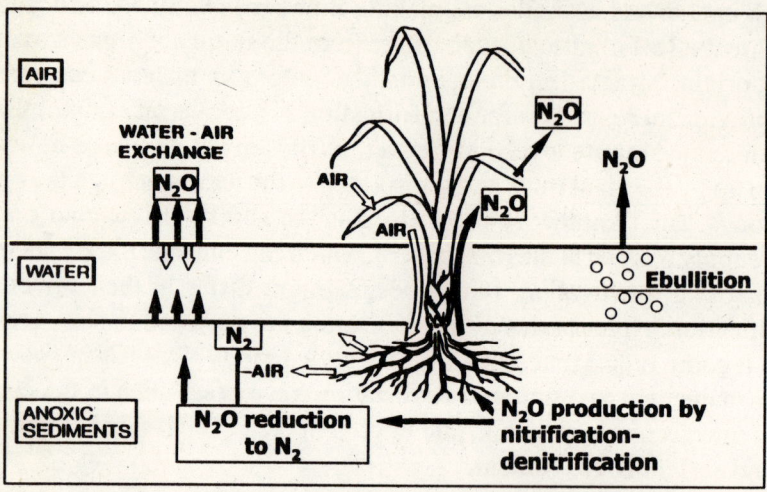

Figure 5: Nitrous oxide production and emission in a rice field: A schematic representation.

transport nitrous oxide from the rhizosphere to the atmosphere. Ebullition of nitrous oxide trapped inside soil is a possible mechanism of its release to the atmosphere. The ebullition process is influenced by many factors like wind speed, water temperature, solar radiation, water level, local water table and atmospheric pressure. In aerobic soils, diffusion plays an important role in transportation of nitrous oxide. However, in waterlogged soils, its role is restricted as diffusion of gases in water is 10^4-times slower than in air, so that the exchange of gases almost stops.

ESTIMATES OF NITROUS OXIDE EMISSION FROM SOIL

The methodologies adopted for nitrous oxide collection at field levels are not yet precise and hence, there are considerable uncertainties in the nitrous oxide estimates. With the advent of sensitive nitrous oxide detection equipment, it is now possible to measure nitrous oxide production directly in the field. Inter-Governmental Panel on Climate Change (IPCC, 1996) reported that the total global emission of nitrous oxide from soils is 5–17 Tg N_2O-N yr^{-1} (Table 1). Estimated anthropogenic sources of nitrous oxide, given in Table 2, shows that agriculture is the most important source of

Table 1. Sources and sinks of nitrous oxide

Source	N_2O-N $(Tg\,yr^{-1})$
Natural	
Oceans	1.4-2.6
Tropical Soils	
Wet forests	2.2-3.7
Dry savannas	0.5-2.0
Temperate Soils	
Forests	0.05-2.0
Grasslands	not estimated
Cultivated soils	0.3-5.0
Biomass burning	0.2-1.0
Stationary combustions	0.1-0.3
Mobile sources	0.2-0.6
Adipic acid production	0.4-0.6
Nitric acid production	0.1-0.3
Total	**5.2-17.0**
Sinks	
Photolysis in stratosphere	7-13
Removal by soils	not estimated
Atmospheric increase	3-4.5

Source: IPCC (1996)

Table 2. Anthropogenic sources of nitrous oxide

Source	N_2O-N $(Tg\,yr^{-1})$
Cultivated soil	3.5
Biomass burning	0.5
Industrial sources	1.3
Cattle and feed lots	0.4
Total	5.7

Source: IPCC (1996)

nitrous oxide emission. As a part global N-cycle (Figure 6), several biotic and abiotic components of the earth contribute to nitrous oxide emission. The major contributors are N fertilizer use, fertilizer production, biomass burning, livestock and industry. Various researchers have indicated that

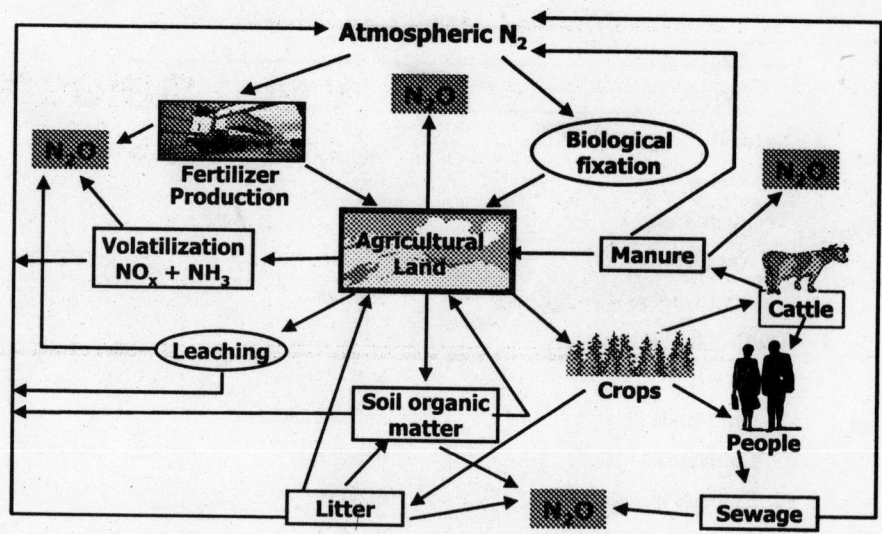

Figure 6: N-cycle and its relation with nitrous oxide emission
(*Source:* Mosier *et al.*, 1998).

emission ranging from <0.001 to 1 kg N_2O-N $ha^{-1}d^{-1}$ are obtained depending on nitrogen fertilization rate, source of nitrogen applied, soil-water content, tillage practices and the prevailing soil temperature. Nitrous oxide emission from different land-use types has been presented in Table 3.

MODELLING NITROUS OXIDE EMISSION FROM SOIL

Quantification of nitrous oxide emission from soil is needed for global modelling studies in the context of ecosystem modification and climate change. Estimates of nitrous oxide emission from soil have been made through field experiments by different researchers. However, these estimates can only partly be extrapolated to farmers' fields and regional scale because of the existence of much broader range of soils, climatic and agronomic conditions. Therefore, estimates of nitrous oxide emission should be based on more generic, quantitative approaches, such as modelling taking into account the climate, soil and cropping variables.

A number of models, for example, CASA (Potter *et al.*, 1993), CENTURY (Parton *et al.*, 1996), ExpertN (Baladioli *et al.*, 1994), Hole-in-the-Pipe (Firestone and Davidson, 1989), NLOOS (Riley and Matson, 1989) and DNDC (Li, 2000) have been developed for N_2O emissions. Some of these process-based models are not yet at a stage where their predictive ability is satisfactory. The input requirements of most of these models are very high and are not easily available. The models have hardly been used in tropical regions. Therefore, there is a need to develop a

Table 3. Nitrous oxide emission from different land-use types

Land-use type	Soil texture	Soil organic C (%)	Fertilizer type	N level (kg ha^{-1})	N$_2$O-N emission (g ha^{-1} day^{-1})	Country
Soil	Medium	2.5	Ammonium	180	31.4	USA
Soil	Fine	4.6	Ammonium	250	107.9	USA
Soil	Medium	2.5	Anhydrous ammonia	180	4.6	USA
Grass	Medium	1.9	Ammonium nitrate	100	24.3	Denmark
Grass	Medium	2.3	Calcium nitrate	400	16.4	UK
Grass	Medium	4.0	Calcium nitrate	400	21.9	UK
Corn	Medium	1.0	Urea	140	29.4	USA
Corn	Fine	1.0	Manure/Urea	273	14.2	USA
Barley	Medium	1.7	Ammonium nitrate	112	6.7	USA
Barley	Medium	1.7	Ammonium nitrate	224	9.2	USA
Wheat			Ammonium nitrate	175	3.5	USA
Wheat			Ammonium nitrate	175	6.5	USA
Rye	Medium		Ammonium nitrate	80	1.6	USA
Rye	Medium		Ammonium nitrate	80	7.9	USA
Tobacco	Medium		Ammonium nitrate	410	68.3	USA
Tobacco	Medium		Green manure		8.8	USA
Cauliflower	Medium		Urea	528	72.9	USA
Cauliflower	Medium		Urea	528	80.0	USA
Rice	Fine	1.69	Urea	120	1.3	Philippines
Rice	Fine	0.45	Urea	120	6.9	India
Wheat	Fine	0.45	Urea	120	6.2	India

Source: Pathak (1999)

process-based model with fewer input requirements for estimation of nitrous oxide emission from soil under field crops in tropical regions.

STRATEGIES TO REDUCE THE EMISSION OF NITROUS OXIDE FROM SOIL

Appropriate crop management practices, which lead to increased N-use efficiency and yield, hold the key to reduce nitrous oxide emissions. Plant uptake of N can be improved and total N losses can be reduced by deep fertilizer placement and by banding fertilizer within the crop rows. Nitrogen-use efficiency can also be promoted by applying fertilizer close to the time of its need by the crop, and by using soil and plant tests prior to fertilization to determine the amount of fertilizer needed by the plant. Cover crops can also keep available soil N away from the microbes responsible for nitrous oxide production. Mitigation strategies for nitrous oxide emission from soil have been discussed in Chapter 10.

The foregoing discussion suggests that though considerable work has been done on nitrous oxide emission from soil but the available information is inadequate for different land-use types with varying soil management. Simple and accurate technologies need to be developed for quantifying nitrous oxide emission. Simulation models should be developed to estimate nitrous oxide emission from various land-use types at field, regional and national scales. The relative contributions of denitrification and nitrification towards the emission of nitrous oxide are to be estimated. The use of biochemicals for controlling nitrous oxide emissions and non-target effects should be studied and their economic feasibility evaluated. Field measurements have to be conducted for precise estimations through simulation models.

CHAPTER 4

Carbon dioxide emission from soil

H. PATHAK, MONIKA RASTOGI, H.K. RAI *and* ANIL SHARMA

*"The world is not growing worse and it is not growing better – it is
just turning around as usual."—Finley Peter Dunne*

CARBON DIOXIDE (CO_2) is the most important greenhouse gas accounting for 60% of the total greenhouse effect. The concentration of carbon dioxide in the atmosphere has increased from 290 ppmV at the beginning of the industrial revolution to 356 ppmV at present and is increasing
at the rate of 1.5 ppmV annually. At present, the main anthropogenic
source of carbon dioxide emission is fossil fuel burning but its release from
the terrestrial biota, including soil emission and clearing and burning of
forests, has contributed significantly to its present concentration in the atmosphere. It has been estimated that changes in land-use from 1850 to
1990 have resulted in cumulative emissions of 122 ± 40 Gt (1 Gt = 10^9
tonnes) carbon which accounts for one half of the worldwide carbon dioxide increase (Houghton, 1995).

The prediction of global climate change has focused attention on soil as
major source and sink for atmospheric CO_2. Besides disturbing the earth's
heat budget, emission of carbon dioxide from soil diminishes soil organic
carbon and soil fertility and productivity. This is also happening due to the
introduction of intensive agriculture and limited recycling of organic residues in soil. As a result, organic carbon content of soils in the tropical regions, where temperature is high, has gone down, reducing soil fertility.
However, it is generally considered that emission of CO_2 from soil and its
uptake by plants during photosynthesis is a self-sustaining system. This
means that for a steady state ecosystem, the quantity of carbon released
from the soil as CO_2 during the year is roughly the same as is fixed by
plants through photosynthesis. But, the actual seasonal pattern of carbon
dioxide evolution from the soil surface and its uptake by the crop commu-

nity may be different. Though agriculture contributes to atmospheric carbon dioxide, it has the potential to act as a sink also. The potential for agriculture to sequester carbon comes mainly from the build up of organic matter (carbon) in agricultural soils. The process of photosynthesis is a major sink for atmospheric CO_2. The non-harvested plant biomass is returned to the soil and contributes to the carbon sequestration. In the final analysis, soils are generally considered to be a source of CO_2, unless the C-inputs outweigh the outputs, which is not usually the case in conventionally tilled low to medium input production systems. This chapter deals with (i) the processes and factors affecting CO_2 formation and emission from soil, (ii) estimates of CO_2 emission from agriculture, and (iii) strategies to sequester C in soil.

CARBON DIOXIDE AS A NATURAL GAS

An English scientist and clergyman, Joseph Priestly, first discovered carbon dioxide (O═C═O), which is a colourless gas with faintly pungent odour and acidic taste with molecular weight 44. It is quite soluble in water. Carbon dioxide occurs naturally in the earth's atmosphere where it serves as an essential plant nutrient and important determinant of the earth's thermal balance. Carbon dioxide being transparent to visible light and partially opaque to the infra-red, interferes with the earth's energy budget. The atmospheric abundance, life-time, sources and sinks of CO_2 are given in Chapter 1 along with other greenhouse gases.

CARBON RESERVES IN THE EARTH

Principal global carbon pools in the earth and fluxes between them have been presented in Figure 1. The largest reservoirs of carbon in the earth are the deep oceans, which hold 50-times more carbon (37000 Gt C) (1 Gt =

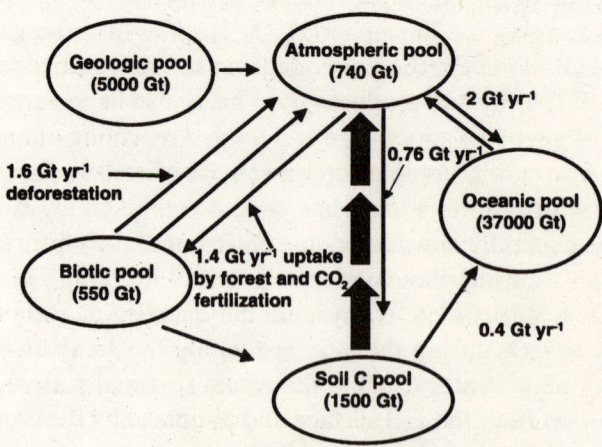

Figure 1: Principal global C pool and fluxes between them.

10^9 ton) than the atmosphere (740 Gt C) (Houghton, 1995). The soils contain about twice (1500 Gt C) as much carbon as the atmosphere. The amount of carbon stored in soils under agriculture is approximately 170 Gt C (Paustian *et al.,* 2000) and vegetation contains 550 Gt C. Forests hold almost half of the world's terrestrial carbon. Soils and vegetation together exchange 100 Gt C yr^{-1} with the atmosphere, while soil respiration alone contributes 50-75 Gt C yr^{-1} (Kicklighter *et al.*, 1994). The net efflux of carbon to the atmosphere from various reservoirs is 5.6 to 6.0 Gt C yr^{-1} (Sundquist, 1994). The total C lost as a result of cultivation worldover has been estimated to be 54 Gt with a maximum observed in temperate grassland and tropical forest soils and the least in Andosols (Mosier, 1998).

The carbon stocks of Indian soils have been calculated using organic carbon data of soil profiles from various sites (Gupta and Rao, 1994). The current total stocks are estimated to be 24.3 Gt of carbon (Table 1), which is 1.6-1.8% of the carbon stored in the world's soils.

Table 1. Current and potential stocks of carbon in Indian soils

Soils	Area (m ha)	Percentage of area	Carbon stocks (Gt)	Carbon carrying capacity (Gt)
Red loamy	50.5	15.3	4.20	6.01
Red and lateritic	20.8	6.3	1.99	3.22
Red and yellow	13.3	4.0	0.60	0.85
Shallow and medium	33.0	10.0	2.71	3.57
Medium and deep black	26.6	8.1	2.45	3.30
Mixed red and black	39.2	11.9	4.75	6.51
Coastal alluvium-derived	8.1	2.5	0.43	0.70
Alluvium-derived	66.1	20.1	3.77	5.65
Desert (and saline) soils	29.6	9.0	0.84	1.30
Brown and red hill	8.0	2.4	1.04	1.68
Shallow and skeletal	15.6	4.7	0.19	0.28
Brown forests and podzolic	17.7	5.4	1.36	1.87
Total	**328.5**	**99.7**	**24.33**	**34.93**

Source: Gupta and Rao (1994)

MECHANISM OF CARBON DIOXIDE EMISSION FROM SOIL

Carbon dioxide emission from soil represents the sum total of all soil metabolic functions in which carbon dioxide is produced (Figure 2). It includes microbial respiration, root respiration, faunal respiration and chemical oxidation of carbonaceous compounds. Release of CO_2 from soil takes place by bacterial, fungal, algal, and protozoan respirations, primarily at the soil surface or within a thin upper layer where the bulk of the plant residue is concentrated. The rate of CO_2 emission varies under different climatic conditions. Tropical soils show higher emission rates compared to the soils of temperate regions because of higher and longer thermal regime. The sources and sinks of CO_2 in agro-ecosystem are reasonably well known, but the magnitude of the fluxes is uncertain. The carbon dioxide concentration in soil is much higher than that in the atmosphere because of the continued generation of CO_2 by biological processes. The general levels of soil carbon dioxide under aerobic conditions are approximately 6000 ppm where active microbial or plant growth occurs. Under the waterlogged conditions, soil CO_2 levels of 10,000–30,000 ppm are considered as average. So the variability in soil water-content is probably one of the most confounding factors affecting CO_2 emission. In the following section factors influencing CO_2 emission from soil have been discussed.

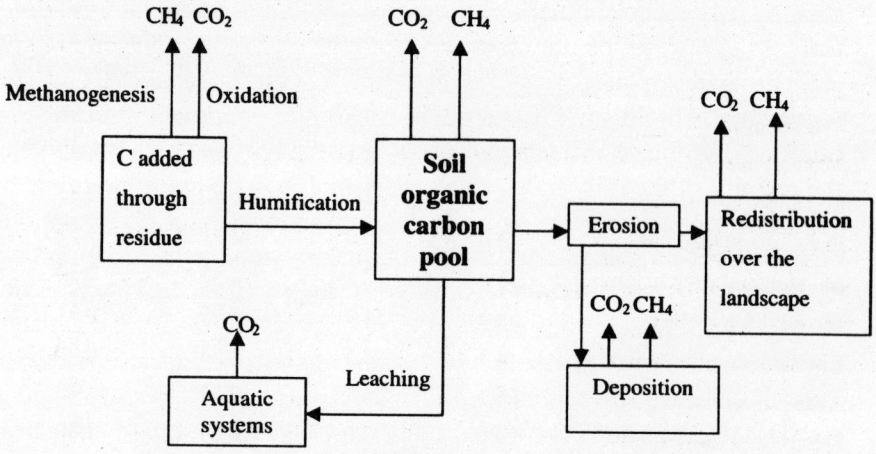

Figure 2: Process affecting soil carbon dynamics (Lal, 2002).

FACTORS AFFECTING CARBON DIOXIDE EMISSION FROM SOIL

Several studies have shown that factors such as soil temperature, texture, moisture, pH, available C and N, etc. influence CO_2 production and emission from soil.

Temperature

Temperature has a marked effect on CO_2 evolution from soil by influencing root and soil respirations. There exists a strong positive relationship between

CO_2 evolution and mean daily soil temperature. At high temperatures (> 40°C), partial inhibition of respiration occurs due to inactivation of the biological oxidation systems. Evolution of CO_2 from the surface of soil cultivated to wheat varies from 4 to 8 g m^{-2} d^{-1} in spring but in winter when soil temperature is below 5°C, its evolution is less than 1 g m^{-2} d^{-1}. In spring, as the ambient temperature increases, CO_2 production in the soil profile increases rapidly by 2.0 to 3.2%. In a study, maximum carbon dioxide production rate was noted in mid July (19 g m^{-2} d^{-1}), which is attributed to the increasing role of soil respiration, root activity and organic matter decomposition with the increase in temperature (Buyanovsky *et al.*, 1986). The rate of organic matter decomposition in tropical rain forests is much higher than that in the arctic region due to the influence of temperature on CO_2 emission.

Moisture

Besides temperature, soil moisture-content also affects soil respiration and hence, CO_2 evolution. These two factors are interdependent with the influence of soil water-content being stronger at higher temperatures. Below the optimum water-content for microbial activity, increasing soil moisture content results in increasing carbon dioxide evolution but above this level, increase in soil moisture reduces CO_2 evolution. Periodic drying and wetting of the soil also influences CO_2 evolution. When the soil is rewetted, the activity of the microbes, which are found in the latent state in the dry soil, increases accompanied by release of air trapped in the soil pores. This contributes to an increase in CO_2 evolution on rewetting the soil. Similarly, drought tends to reduce and rewetting increases carbon dioxide emission. Under dry soil conditions, soil respiration is higher during the day than at night. It is similar at day and night when the soil is wet due to reduction in variability in the soil temperature. The drainage of water-logged soil increases CO_2 emission. The amount of CO_2 released from rice fields during the drying period is double than during the flooding. These differences in the CO_2 budget are mainly due to increase in its emission from the soil surface under drained conditions, resulting from the removal of the diffusion barrier caused by floodwater.

Soil texture

Soil-texture affects the spread of microbial propagules and the growth of bacteria and fungi and thus formation of CO_2. The rate of carbon dioxide evolution is greater from heavy soils, which has a higher organic C content than light soils, although the percentage of C lost from heavy soil is less than from coarser soils. Even under fallow conditions, the clay loam shows higher CO_2 evolution than sandy and loam soils.

Soil pH

Hydrogen ion activity (pH) of soil has a marked effect on the growth of bacteria, fungi and soil fauna. In soils having pH 3.0, 2- to 12-fold less CO_2 concentration has been observed than at pH 4.0 (Sitaula *et al.*, 1995). It is due to the adverse effect of low pH on soil microbial activity, which lowers respiration rate and consequently there is less CO_2 evolution. At higher pH, increase in CO_2 evolution is observed up to pH 7.0, beyond which also adverse effect is observed. For example, at pH 8.7, CO_2 emission was found to be reduced by 18% and at pH 10.0 by 83% compared to that at pH 7.0 (Rao and Pathak, 1996).

Salinity

Excessive amount of salts have adverse effect on physical and chemical properties of soil and microbiological processes. These include effect on C and N mineralization and soil enzyme activities, which are crucial for decomposition of organic matter and evolution of CO_2. A progressive decrease in CO_2 evolution occurs with increase in salinity. Carbon mineralization is almost similar in soils up to the electrical conductivity (EC) value 26 d S m^{-1}, but gets drastically reduced at higher EC (Pathak and Rao, 1998). Organic manure amendment, however, increases the biological evolution of CO_2 from saline soils, except at a very high salinity.

Atmospheric pressure

The atmospheric pressure is directly related with emission of CO_2; its decrease triggers the release of CO_2 from the soil, thereby enhancing CO_2 emission.

Organic manure amendment

Application of manures to soil can also increase CO_2 emission. The soluble organic carbon in soil is an immediate source of carbon for soil microorganisms, which in turn emit CO_2. Therefore, addition of large quantities of readily decomposable organic matter to agricultural soils may contribute significantly to atmospheric CO_2 (Rastogi *et al.*, 2002). Manures including sewage sludge amendment, increase the soil respiration by a factor of 2-3 (Scott *et al.*, 2000). Similarly, incorporation of crop residue increases CO_2 flux but the effect is small compared to mulching of straw. High quality residues, i.e. with high N from grain legumes or fodders, can accelerate the decomposition of soil organic matter because of the availability of additional N to the microbial population.

Fertilizer application

The application of nitrogenous fertilizer affects CO_2 emission directly by providing N to microbes, which, in turn, increase the decomposition of soil organic matter and indirectly, by influencing soil pH, which affects microbial activity. However, reduction in CO_2 emission from soil is observed at very high N application rate due to the reduced microbial respiration by increased acidity. Moreover, increase in the supply of NH_4^+-N to soil reduces the decay of organic matter and CO_2 emission. Application of phosphate and potash increases CO_2 emission from soil. Another source of atmospheric CO_2 usually neglected, is agricultural lime added to counteract the soil acidity. The applied lime dissolves to form HCO_3^- or $CO_3^=$ ions, depending on the acid-base balance of the soil solution, and any CO_2 formed will be released to the atmosphere.

Use of nitrification inhibitors

Nitrification inhibitors, viz. DCD (dicyandiamide), nitrapyrin, sodium thiosulphate, 2-amino-4-chloro–6-methyl-pyrimidine (AM), and acetylene, inhibit the nitrification process where ammonical form of nitrogen is oxidized by microbes to the nitrate form. These chemicals are recommended to increase nitrogen-use efficiency and reduce N-loss through leaching and denitrification. However, these chemicals might also act on those microbes, which are engaged in the oxidation of organic carbon and reduce CO_2 emission. It has been shown that a nitrification inhibitor, encapsulated calcium carbide (a slow release source of acetylene), reduces carbon dioxide emission and appears to be effective in minimizing emission of this greenhouse gas in flooded rice. However, studies on the effect of nitrification inhibitors on carbon dioxide emission is limited and needs detailed investigations.

Crops

The presence of crops influences carbon dioxide production and emission from soil. The production of carbon dioxide is approximately 2- to 3-fold more in cropped soils compared to bare soils. Within different crops also, there is a variability in carbon dioxide production. In an alluvial, sandy loam soil, having pH 7.5 and organic matter 0.66%, planted to wheat and maize crops, CO_2 emissions have been found as 36.7 and 61.7 kg CO_2 ha^{-1} d^{-1}, respectively. Higher CO_2 emission in maize crop is partly attributed to favourable temperature and moisture conditions during its growth (July to October), while a decrease in total soil respiration during the wheat crop is due to lower temperature during November to January.

Tillage

The main source of CO_2 to the atmosphere from cultivated systems is probably through tillage. During a tillage event, soil aggregates are broken, increasing oxygen supply and surface area exposure of organic material. This promotes the decomposition of organic matter. Thus, more CO_2 emission can occur from a tilled than from an undisturbed soil (no till). Low or zero CO_2 fluxes under no-tillage are associated with reduced gas diffusivity and air-filled porosity. Enhancement of C mineralization and its atmospheric fluxes with tillage suggest that tillage intensity should be minimized to reduce C losses from soil.

Soil depth

Soil depth is another factor affecting CO_2 emission and it increases with depth in the soil profile. The maximum emission of CO_2 takes place from the surface layers where greater microbial activity occurs, whereas a general decrease in respiration rate occurs with increase in depth. The top 5-cm of the soil profile contributes 75% of the daily rate of carbon dioxide production, whereas the 5 to 10 cm segment of the profile yields an additional 10% of the daily output, leaving 15% to be accounted for by the deeper layers.

SPATIAL, TEMPORAL AND SEASONAL VARIABILITY IN CARBON DIOXIDE FLUX

Spatial variability of soil respiration may occur at a scale smaller than 15-cm in cropped fields, which is attributed to the contribution of plant roots to soil respiration, as maximum soil respiration during the growing season coincides with the period of maximum growth. There are considerable variations in CO_2 emission during the different spans of the day and night. For a grassland soil, the average day and night soil respiration rates are 10.36 and 8.64 g CO_2 m^{-2} d^{-1}. This is attributed to a higher soil temperature during the day. The soil temperature, which accounts for the most of the temporal variability on CO_2 efflux, is thus by far the most influential factor controlling soil respiration rate. Besides the diurnal variation, there is seasonal variation on soil respiration, with maximum soil respiration during the growing season coinciding with period of maximum growth of crops. Seasonal CO_2 flux is maximum in spring followed by in summer, autumn and winter. In spring, neither temperature is limiting nor moisture but in summer, moisture becomes limiting and in winters, the limiting factor is temperature.

MITIGATION OF CARBON DIOXIDE
EMISSION FROM AGRICULTURE

The mitigation of CO_2 evolution from agriculture can be achieved by increasing carbon sequestration in soil through manipulation of soil pH, soil water-content, temperature, setting aside surplus agriculture land, and restoration of soil carbon on degraded land. A detailed account of carbon sequestration in soil has been presented in Chapter 9 and only a brief account has been presented here.

Soil management strategies for carbon sequestration include three approaches. Firstly, management of soils to maintain existing levels of soil organic matter such as reduced tillage and no tillage practices. Second approach is to manage carbon-degraded soils to restore depleted soil organic matter levels. Wastelands in India are over 100 m ha of which 70% are carbon-degraded. These carbon-depleted soils have relatively high potential for accumulating organic carbon in vegetation and soil if suitable trees are grown along with the proper soil conservation measures. Since wastelands like salt-affected soils represent a great potential for sequestering carbon, it is desirable to promote agro-forestry in these soils. The third approach is to manage soils to enlarge soil organic matter pools by improving soil fertility. Soil processes could be managed so that litter production exceeds decomposition. Such an approach of increasing carrying capacity of soils is difficult as it is determined by factors such as climate that cannot be managed. Another approach could be to increase passive or inert fraction of soil organic pool. This implies taking soil organic carbon out of humification-mineralization cycle. This can be achieved through the increase of sub-soil organic carbon and micro aggregation. Subsoil organic carbon can be increased by growing deep rooted plants, deep ploughing while micro aggregation can be increased by using soil conditioners, long-chain polymers and earthworms.

CHAPTER 5

Ammonia volatilization from soil

H. PATHAK, BIDISHA BANERJEE *and* SONALI MAZUMDAR

"Nature encourages no looseness, pardons no errors."
—Ralph Waldo Emerson

THE GREEN REVOLUTION IN INDIA owes a considerable part of its success to fertilizer application and nitrogen (N) is the most widely used fertilizer nutrient. The consumption of fertilizer was 0.78 million tons in 1965, which is 16.7 million tons today and more than 65 per cent of it is nitrogenous fertilizer. Since, nutrient use is sub-optimal in many regions, increase in fertilizer consumption could be a strategy for more food production. But concerns have been expressed about the adverse impact of fertilizers on the environment. This makes sense as N-use efficiency of crops seldom exceeds 50 per cent and a considerable portion is lost from the soil-plant-system through leaching, run-off, denitrification, and volatilization and pollutes the soil, water, and air, which are the vital resources of nature (Figure 1, Chapter 3). There is a growing evidence that due to the imbalanced use of fertilizers, physical and chemical properties of soil are deteriorating, water is being polluted with nitrate, and the atmosphere is being enriched with nitrous oxide (N_2O), posing a threat of global warming and ozone layer depletion due to over reliance on mineral fertilizer. It is, therefore, important to understand the fate of fertilizers when added to soil.

Ammonia (NH_3) volatilization is one of the important loss mechanisms affecting the N-use efficiency. The magnitude of NH_3 loss can be as high as 90% when N is applied to the surface of sandy soils with very low buffering capacity. High NH_3 loss from soil highlights the importance of NH_3 volatilization as a loss mechanism. Volatilization of NH_3 is also a cause of environmental pollution. From the atmosphere, NH_3 is washed out by clouds and redeposit on the terrestrial ecosystem and then oxidized to N_2O, a greenhouse gas and also responsible for destruction of ozone layer. The chapter presents (i) sources ad sinks of ammonia, (ii) the mechanism and factors affecting volatilization loss from soil, and (iii) strategies to reduce NH_3 volatilization losses.

SOURCES AND SINKS OF ATMOSPHERIC AMMONIA

The important sources and sinks for NH_3 in the atmosphere are depicted in Figure 1. The sources include ammonium or ammonium forming fertilizers, industrial pollutants, animal wastes, and shallow natural or manmade water bodies. Small amounts of NH_3 are also lost from decaying plant residues and maturing plants. The major sources of NH_3, however, are urea and ammonium-based fertilizers, animal and sewage wastes, and soil contributing about 55% of the anthropogenic NH_3 released annually to the atmosphere. This release of NH_3 represents an enormous loss of nutrients and energy from agricultural systems.

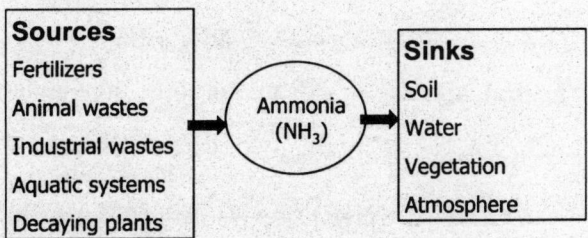

Figure 1: Potential sources and sinks for atmospheric NH_3

MECHANISMS OF AMMONIA VOLATILIZATION FROM SOIL

Ammonia volatilization from soil has been of research interest since the use of commercial N fertilizer on a large-scale following World War II. Until about 20 years ago, NH_3 volatilization was studied only under controlled laboratory conditions. Recent research under field conditions has required development of methods of measuring NH_3 losses under these conditions and has led to a better understanding of NH_3 volatilization.

The reaction mechanism by which NH_3 loss occurs from fertilizer N applied to soil depends on the kind of N compound and the chemical characteristics of the soils. Some reactions are purely chemical and rapid, whereas NH_3 loss from urea depends on microbiological transformation and leads to slower losses initially. The overall rates of NH_3 volatilization from urea is controlled by different steps shown in the chain in Scheme 1.

Ammonia volatilization from urea occurs in acid, neutral, and alkaline

$$\text{Urea} \longrightarrow NH_4^+\text{-Soil} \rightleftharpoons NH_3\text{-Soil} \rightleftharpoons NH_3\text{-Gas} \rightleftharpoons NH_3\text{-Atmosphere}$$

$$\downarrow$$

$$NO_3^-\text{-Soil}$$

Scheme 1. Different Steps of NH₃ Volatilization.

or calcareous soils. In moist acid soils, urea [$CO(NH_2)_2$] is hydrolyzed by urease enzyme to ammonium (NH_4^+) ions [Eq. (1)]:

$$CO(NH_2)_2 + 2H_2O + H^+ \longrightarrow 2NH_4^+ + HCO_3^- \qquad (1)$$

In this reaction, H^+ in acid soils are consumed and thus an alkaline condition (pH above 7) in immediate vicinity of urea droplets is induced temporarily. Under alkaline conditions, a part of NH_4^+ ions form free NH_3:

$$NH_4^+ \longrightarrow NH_3 + H^+ \qquad (2)$$

In moist neutral, alkaline or calcareous soils, urea undergoes hydrolysis:

$$CO(NH_2)_2 + 2H_2O \xrightarrow{\text{Urease}} (NH_4)_2CO_3 \qquad (3)$$

$$(NH_4)_2CO_3 \longrightarrow 2NH_3 + CO_2 + H_2O \qquad (4)$$

A part of this NH_3 can volatilize, and the other part dissolves in soil water to yield ammonium hydroxide:

$$NH_3 + H_2O \rightleftharpoons NH_4OH \qquad (5)$$

Ammonium hydroxide increases the soil pH. Moreover, it dissociates to yield NH_4^+ and OH^- ions as shown in Eq. (6):

$$NH_4OH \rightleftharpoons NH_4^+ + OH^- \qquad (6)$$

Under alkaline conditions, a part of NH_4^+ ions is converted to free NH_3:

$$NH_4^+ \longrightarrow NH_3 + H^+ \qquad (7)$$

Most of the NH_3 volatilization losses take place within two weeks of urea application. The losses are generally less in the beginning due to the delay in the hydrolysis of urea. The overlying water reduces the rate of urea hydrolysis because of little urease activity in the floodwater and the transfer of dissolved urea to the soil surface before it can be hydrolyzed. However, in well-drained soils, the loss is the maximum during the first three days after N application. The loss decreases with time thereafter. It has been reported that most of the ammonia volatilization losses occur within seven days after fertilizer application. Band placement of urea reduces the loss to below 5% of applied N. When urea super granules are used, this loss is reduced to about 3%.

FACTORS AFFECTING NH_3 VOLATILIZATION

The extent of volatilization loss depends on several of soil, plant, and climatic factors. Ammonia losses from field may be erratic because of such parameters as oscillating temperatures, changes in humidity, variable wind speed, rainfall, and other environmental factors. It is possible that no serious losses of ammonia may occur for several days and then a severe loss may happen when environmental conditions are favourable for NH_3 volatilization. Although the soil properties largely determine the potential for NH_3 loss, it is the environmental condition that determines the actual magnitude of loss under field conditions.

Moisture regime

The variability in soil-water content is probably one of the most confounding factors affecting NH_3 volatilization. Adequate surface-soil moisture has to exist to permit optimum rates of urea hydrolysis and subsequent transformations of N. Ammonia volatilization losses in soil increases with increase in soil water-content, from air dry to flooding. But, as the depth of floodwater increases, volatilization loss is decreased due to decrease in NH_4^+-N concentration of the floodwater. For maximum NH_3 losses, the soil water-content must be at or near field capacity at the time of fertilizer application. Azolla, generally growing in flooded rice fields, reduces the NH_3 volatilization (Vlek and Henning, 1995). This reduction in NH_3 volatilization is largely related to the decrease of the floodwater pH by azolla; whose absence may take pH values to 9 and 10.

Source of N

Amount of N lost by volatilization depends on the type of fertilizer used. The differences in NH_3 volatilization from different fertilizers are due to their properties like the form of N, associated anions, and acidic or alkaline nature of the fertilizers. Fertilizers with high inherent alkalinity such as urea or aqueous ammonia, if applied improperly, lead to extensive NH_3 losses, irrespective of soil pH. On the contrary, acid-producing fertilizers like ammonium sulphate emit less NH_3. The NH_3 losses from different fertilizers have been found in the following order: Diammonium phosphate

(DAP) > urea > ammonium sulphate > calcium ammonium nitrate > ammonium nitrate > ammonium chloride. Coated-urea fertilizers like neem-coated and polymer-coated urea as well as urea super granule help in reducing NH_3 emissions from soils. The form of a fertilizer also affects NH_3 loss. When broadcast, liquid forms tend to lose more NH_3 than dry forms.

Method of application

Maximum NH_3 loss occurrs when N fertilizers are broadcast on the soil surface compared to placement or incorporation in soil. The loss is much less due to topdressing of N compared to basal application because of large crop canopy.

Soil pH and buffering capacity

Activity of H^+ ions (pH) in soil largely determines the ratio of NH_3 to NH_4^+ ion in soil solution. Hence, soil pH is an important factor influencing NH_3 volatilization loss and with increase in pH, the loss increases. Higher volatilization loss is observed in calcareous and sodic soils due to high pH of floodwater. Higher NH_3 losses with urea than ammonium sulphate are also due to increase in pH in floodwater with urea application. Ammonium sulphate lowers the pH of the water below 7 and reduces the NH_3 loss. The H^+ buffering capacity of soil is more important than the initial soil pH in determining NH_3 loss potential; it decreases with increase in H^+ buffering capacity.

Cation exchange capacity

The cation exchange capacity (CEC) of a soil is important for NH_3 loss because it provides a mechanism by which NH_4^+ ions are removed from soil solution, thereby reducing the total amount of ammonical N in the soil solution, which is subject to volatilization. There is a negative correlation between CEC and NH_3 loss and it appears that a minimum CEC of 25 c mol (p^+) kg^{-1} is required to substantially reduce NH_3 volatilization (Lyster *et al.*, 1980).

Concentration of NH_4^+ ions in soil solution

The rate of ammonia volatilization is directly related to the concentration of NH_4^+ ions in soil solution and therefore to its pH and the loss is correlated with HCO_3^- and NH_4^+-N concentrations in floodwater. In rice fields, the high floodwater NH_4^+-N following N application along with high temperature creates a favourable environment for ammonia loss to occur.

Temperature

Under controlled condition, NH_3 loss due to volatilization increases with rise in temperature as the latter affects chemical and biochemical reactions, specially urease activity in soil given adequate moisture to ensure complete and rapid urea hydrolysis. In a majority of field studies, maximum NH_3 loss was reported to occur between 10.00 and 12.00 hours of the day (Hargrove *et al.,* 1987). Generally, this corresponds to a time when soil temperature is increasing but is not the maximum. The reason for maximum NH_3 loss not occurring at maximum temperature is probably that the soil becomes drier at this temperature. For maximum NH_3 losses, the soil water-content must be at or near field capacity. If the soil surface dries but is not rewetted by dew or rainfall, NH_3 loss is reduced because of insufficient moisture for the necessary biochemical and chemical reactions.

Wind speed

Under field conditions, volatilization loss increases linearly with wind speed as the latter carries away the NH_3 formed creating the concentration gradient, which favours higher volatilization (Fillery *et al.,* 1984). However, air-exchange rate in the field does not limit NH_3 volatilization, since even on windless rainy days, the rate of NH_3 volatilization is found to be high.

Plant

In the plants NH_3 can be produced and released to the atmosphere and this process is favoured by high temperature and transpiration. The NH_3 losses from soybean foliage have been reported as high as 45 kg N ha^{-1}. The release of NH_3 from the leaves or its absorption by leaves depends on the partial pressure of NH_3 in the atmosphere. Plants, on the other hand can influence NH_3 loss by removing N from soil, influencing urease activity and modifying the soil environment. Ammonia volatilization loss varies with growth stages of rice. Compared to the seedling stage, the NH_3 volatilization loss is much less when a fertilizer is applied at panicle initiation stage, since the demand of N by the crops is very high during this period.

Organic matter amendment

Amendment of soil with organic matter in the form of farmyard manure (FYM) reduces the volatilization losses of NH_3. The NH_3 volatilization has been found to reduce from 20% in the unamended soil to 13.7, 12.0, 6.3, and 6.2% with the addition of cowpea, sesbania, wheat straw, and rice straw in the soil, respectively. But when urea is applied at 10-cm soil depth addition of organic matter does not have any significant effect on NH_3 loss. It is observed that in wetland rice ecosystems, ammonia fluxes are considerably lower with green manure than with urea. This is due to increased pCO_2 concentration in floodwater with green manure incorporation in the wetland soil that lowers the pH of the floodwater thereby reducing NH_3 loss. On the other hand the soils that have inadequate supplies of urease for maximum ammonia loss, the volatilization may increase upon addition of organic matter.

Nitrification inhibitor

Since nitrification inhibitors retard nitrification, ammonium N can accumulate and result in a higher soil pH, ooth of which are conducive to ammonia volatilization. The volatilization losses of ammonia with nitrification inhibitors can be reduced by incorporation of the fertilizer N. Another possibility of reducing volatilization is the use of dual-purpose (nitrification inhibitor and urease inhibitor) compounds such as thiophosphoryl triamide (Radel *et al.*, 1992).

ESTIMATES OF NH₃ VOLATILZATION LOSS

Estimates of ammonia emission from various land-use types in India are given in Table 1. These values vary from 0.98 to 25.8 kg ha^{-1}, depending upon the soil type, crop and fertilizer material. In a study at IARI, New Delhi, the loss of N as NH_3 from the rice–wheat system was in the range of 38.6 kg ha^{-1} from the unfertilized soil to 69.0 kg ha^{-1} with urea plus DCD treatment (Banerjee *et al.*, 2002). Daily emission of NH_3-N was as high as 0.45 kg ha^{-1} d^{-1} in rice and 0.5 kg ha^{-1} d^{-1} in wheat. Substitution of 50% N provided by urea by FYM reduces the NH_3-N emission by 10% in rice and wheat as compared to only urea treatment. The application of nitrification inhibitor, dicyandiamide (DCD), has been found to increase NH_3-N emission by 7% in wheat with no effect in rice. The annual emission of ammonia from fertilized soils in India is estimated to be 1.175 million tons with urea alone contributing 1.103 million tons (Table 2).

STRATEGIES TO REDUCE NH₃ VOLATILIZATION

The management practices that decrease the pH of soil or irrigation water, increase CEC, or move the fertilizer deeper into the soil profile (i.e. injecting fertilizer or irrigation after application) decrease NH_3 losses. Management factors like sub-surface application of fertilizers, fertilizer modification, etc. can also reduce NH_3 losses by modifying soil properties, urea hy-

Table 1. Volatilization of ammonia from various land-use types and locations of India

Location	Crop	Soil organic C (%)	pH	Texture*	N added (kg ha^{-1})	N source†	Volatilization loss (kg ha^{-1})
‡IARI, New Delhi	Rice	0.48	7.7	SCL	120	Urea	10.08
IARI, New Delhi	Rice	0.48	7.7	SCL	120	USG	3.96
IARI, New Delhi	Wheat	0.41	8.2	L	100	Urea	7.96
Kalyani, West Bengal	Rice	1.23	8.4	SiCL	90	Urea	15.6
Kalyani, West Bengal	Rice	1.23	8.4	SiCL	90	NCU	12
Kalyani, West Bengal	Rice	1.23	8.4	SiCL	90	Urea + GM	7.2
Cuttack, Orissa	Rice	0.70	6.0	SiL	90	Urea	2.86
Pantnagar, Uttaranchal	Rice	—	7.6	—	120	Urea	22.8
Pantnagar, Uttaranchal	Rice	—	7.6	—	120	USG	0.96
Cuttack, Orissa	Rice	0.70	5.6	SCL	80	Urea	5.5
Ujjain, Madhya Pradesh	—	0.45	—	CL	120	Urea	25.8
Ujjain, Madhya Pradesh	—	0.45	—	CL	120	DAP	4.32

*SCL, Sandy clay loam; L, Loam; SiCL, Silty clay loam; SiL, Silty loam; S, Sandy; CL, Clay loam
†USG, Urea super granule; NCU, Neem-coated urea; GM, green manure; DAP, Diammonium phosphate
‡IARI, Indian Agricultural Research Institute
Source: Pathak and Banerjee (2003)

Table 2. Ammonia emissions from different fertilizers in India

Fertilizer	Loss of N as NH$_3$ (%)	NH$_3$ ('000 tons)
Ammonium sulphate	8	11.6
Urea	15	1103.4
Calcium ammonium nitrate	2	4.0
Diammonium phosphate	5	40.3
Ammonium phosphate	2	0.4
Nitrophosphate	3	3.8
NPK complex	4	11.3
Total		1174.8

Source: **Parashar** *et al.* (1998)

drolysis rate, chemical equilibrium, and environmental factors. The following strategies can be adopted for minimization of NH_3 volatilization.

1. Mixing of fertilizer with soil
2. Decreasing the pH of soil or irrigation water using gypsum and pyrite
3. Increasing the CEC by amending soil with manure
4. Drilling the basal dose for upland crop and following broadcast by hoeing
5. Moving the fertilizer deeper into the soil profile by injecting fertilizer or irrigation after application
6. Practicing split application, choosing appropriate time at specified growth stages
7. Using fertilizer formulations such as urea super-granules, coated-fertilizers
8. Practicing the site-specific integrated nutrient management system, and
9. Using urease inhibitors.

Efficient utilization of fertilizer is one of the keys to economic crop yield. This increases N-use efficiency and reduces various losses of N, including volatilization. It is of great importance to optimize the availability of an added N fertilizer to crops not only due to continuous increase in prices of fertilizer but also due to environmental pollution. Volatilization of ammonia from soil is a major loss of N and technologies need to develop to minimize the loss.

CHAPTER 6

Measurement of greenhouse gas emission from soil and developing emission inventories

M.C. JAIN, H. PATHAK *and* ARTI BHATIA

"It stands to the everlasting credit of science that by acting on the human mind it has overcome men's insecurity before himself and before nature."—Albert Einstein

DURING THE LAST TWO decades efforts on the quantitative measurements of the emissions of greenhouse gases from soil have been intensified. One of the major constraints in obtaining reliable gas emission estimates is the lack of standard methodology for measuring these emissions. In this chapter, the methodologies, generally used, for measurement of greenhouse gas emissions from soil have been described and the methodology for preparation of inventory of methane and nitrous oxide emissions has been outlined.

MEASUREMENT OF GREENHOUSE GAS EMISSION

Methane and nitrous oxide

The three methods, generally employed to measure methane and nitrous oxide emissions from soil are:

(a) *Closed Chamber Method*: In this method, gas emissions from soil are usually determined by measuring the short-term buildup of the gas in a sealed enclosure placed over the soil surface.

(b) *Open Chamber Method*: In the open chamber method, air is drawn through the chamber into a collection system that concentrates the gas of interest. Where sensitive analytical capability is not available for direct measurement of the gases and larger sample is required, this method is used. However, normally the widespread availability of gas chromatographs with flame ionization or electron capture detectors make the complex open chamber unnecessary.

(c) *Micrometeorological Method:* This method measures vertical concentration gradients of the gas. However, requirement of expensive equipments and cumbersome sampling and measurement procedures restrict its use for CH_4 and N_2O measurements.

The present discussion will be limited to the closed chamber method only as it is a most widely used method. However, it should be kept in mind that regardless of the gas flux method employed, the measured values can only be properly interpreted if the various soil, plant and climatic factors, which determine the production, consumption and emission of the greenhouse gases, are taken into account. Among these, soil texture, pH, organic matter content, moisture content, nitrate and ammonium content, redox potential, plant cover, and climatic factors such as air temperature, incoming radiation, relative humidity and precipitation are important. Soil physical factors such as bulk density, porosity and pore size distribution are also important in determining the storage and movement of gases in the soil.

Closed chamber method

Gas flux from the soil using closed chambers can be determined by collecting gas samples periodically from the chambers and measuring the change in concentration of a gas with time during the period of linear concentration change. Chambers can be made from material like rigid plastic, metal or acrylic sheets. For collecting gas samples from crop fields, generally, chambers of 50 cm × 30 cm × 100 cm (Figure 1) made of 6-mm acrylic sheets are used. Aluminum channels, used with each chamber, are inserted 10-cm inside the soil and the channels filled with water to make the system air-tight. A battery operated fan is fixed inside the chamber to homogenize the inside air. A thermometer is also inserted to monitor the inside temperature. One 3-way stopcock is fitted at the top of chamber to collect gas samples. The chamber is thoroughly flushed several times with a syringe. Gas samples are drawn with the help of hypodermic needle (Figure 2). After drawing the sample, syringes are made air-tight with a three-way stopcock. Samples of four replications of each treatment are taken from the plots and the average is taken as representative value for the treatment. Head space volume inside the box is recorded, which is used to calculate flux of gas.

To make a flux measurement, the chamber is fixed on the top of the

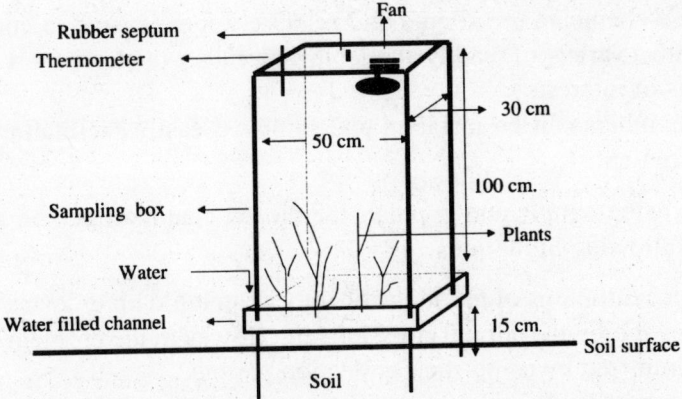

Figure 1: Closed chamber used for gas collection from field

pre-inserted channel and the change in CH_4 or N_2O concentration in the chamber so formed, with time is determined by taking replicate gas samples from the chamber headspace with a syringe (10-20 mL in typical applications; either plastic or greased glass medical syringes fitted with a 2-way or 3-way loop, are satisfactory) and analyzed. Gas samples should be taken from the headspace immediately after sealing and at equal time intervals thereafter over a period not exceeding 2 hours. A minimum of three measurements should be made to check the linearity of concentration increase in the chamber. A departure from a straight line indicates either an inadequately sealed chamber or the decrease in gas concentration gradient between the zone of production in the soil and the chamber atmosphere changes the gas diffusion rate with time. The chamber cover should be removed after the final sample has been taken to minimize the disturbance to environmental conditions within the enclosure formed by the chamber wall.

To transfer gas samples over long distances to the analytical laboratory, evacuated vials fitted with rubber septa (e.g. vacutainers) can be used satisfactorily. The septa on the vials should be cleaned with a detergent and the vials evacuated by a vacuum pump before use. An alternative method is the use of glass serum bottles fitted with butyl rubber stoppers. The vials are taken to the sampling site, and filled with the sample with a syringe. By injecting sufficient sample to achieve an over-pressure, e.g. 10 mL into a 9-mL vial, contamination problems are prevented.

The advantages of the closed chamber method are:

(a) Very small fluxes can be measured.
(b) No extra equipment requiring electrical supply is needed.
(c) There is little disturbance of the site due to the short-time for which the cover has to be placed for each gas flux estimate.

(d) The chambers are simple and relatively inexpensive to construct with a variety of readily available materials, which are inert for the gas of interest.

(e) Chambers can be installed and removed easily facilitating measurement.

Inspite being simple and popular, the closed chamber method suffers from the following limitations.

(a) Concentrations of gas in the chamber can build up to levels where they inhibit the normal emission rate. However, the problem can be minimized by using short collection periods.

(b) Closed chambers alter the atmospheric pressure fluctuations, which are found at the soil surface due to the natural turbulence of air movement. Thus, a closed chamber may underestimate the flux of the gas. The problem may be overcome by an appropriately designed vent, which allows pressure equilibration in and outside the chamber.

(c) Temperature changes in the soil and inside the chamber can occur. However, insulating the chamber and covering it with a reflective material can reduce temperature differences.

For obtaining round the clock emission measurements and to overcome some of the above limitations, automatic sampling devices are very useful. In this device, the air samples from the inner volume of the gas collecting chamber is replaced by a gas flow system providing a periodic sample transfer to the gas chromatograph. Automatic sampling devices require

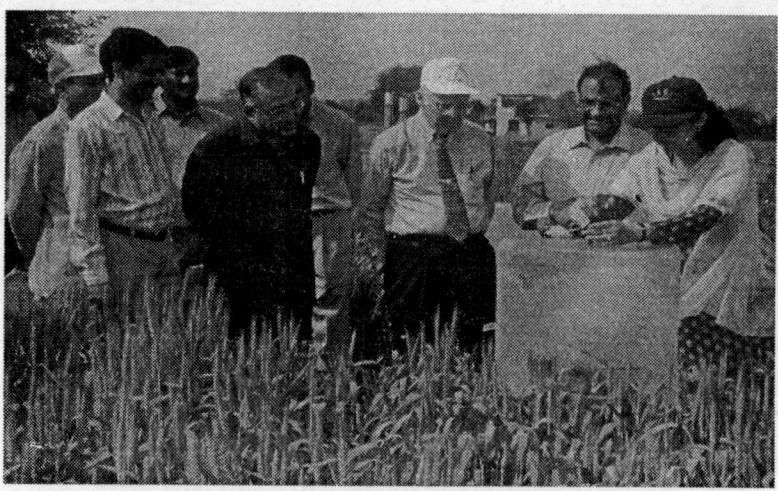

Figure 2: Manual gas sampling from field

greater financial resources and their use is confined to those locations where the laboratory is in the vicinity of the experimental field. The automatic sampling system is extensively used in the long-term field measurements of methane at different experimental stations. The basic components of an automatic sampling system (Figure 3) are: Gas collecting chambers (boxes) equipped with removable covers, gas flow system (tubing, pump), sampling unit, analytical unit (GC and integrator), time control and data acquisition systems. It allows continuous round the clock and simultaneous measurements at several locations for an entire growing season, as is necessary for obtaining data on diurnal and seasonal variations in emission rates under field conditions.

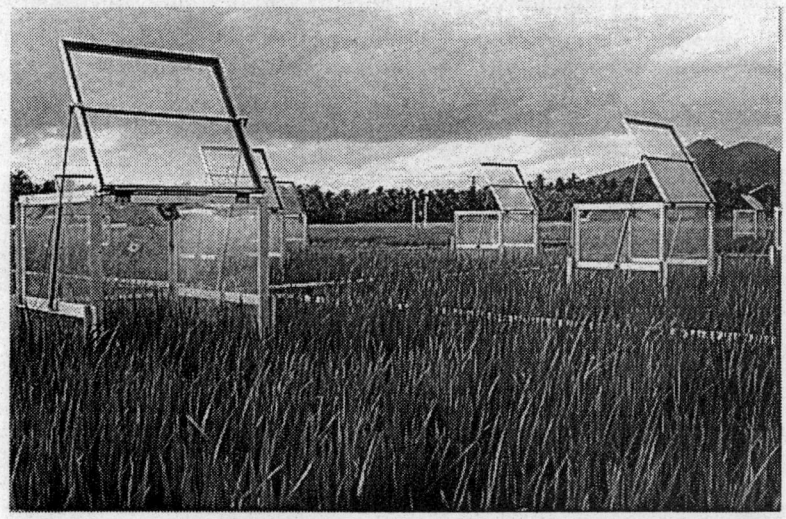

Figure 3: Automated gas sampling from field

ANALYSIS OF GAS SAMPLES

Methane

Before we discuss the analysis of methane, it is necessary to understand the principle under which the equipment flame ionization detector (FID), used for its analysis works. This detector can be used for the detection of substances, which produce ions when heated in an H_2-air flame. The detector is insensitive to permanent gases, water and inorganic ions, which do not ionize at 2100°C. The sample along with the carrier gas (eluent) enters the hydrogen jet via millipore filter. The sample components get ionized to form ions and free electrons on entering the flame at the tip of the jet. The electrons produced are drawn towards the collector. Hence there is a flow of current. The current flow across an external resistor, sensed as a voltage drop, is amplified and displayed on the recorder. The entire assembly is housed in an oven to prevent condensation of water vapour formed as a result of combustion.

Gas samples containing methane are introduced into the gas chromatograph by a syringe fitted with a two-way nylon stopcock through a sampling valve. A gas sample loop of 1 or 2 cm^3 is fitted to the sample valve. It is possible to inject manually, however, the use of a sample loop is to be preferred. The configuration of the valve is normally designed to fit the needs of the user. Methane analysis can be accomplished by various modifications of GC settings and column materials. Each individual setting will have to be optimized empirically in order to achieve a satisfactory separation and detection. Methane can be separated from other gaseous components on a Porapak N column (3-m-long stainless steel or nickel with 3.175-mm outside diameter) maintained at 50°C having a carrier gas flow (helium, nitrogen or argon) of 20 cm^3 min^{-1}. An alternative is the use of a molecular sieve (13 x 60-80 mesh size) as a column material and synthetic air as carrier gas. Methane is detected using a FID maintained at 250°C. The sampling valve can be accentuated manually or time-controlled pneumatically or electronically using computer or GC-contained microprocessor. A GC-computer interface is used to plot and measure the peak area.

Calculation of methane flux

Cross-sectional area of the chamber (m^2)   =   A
Headspace (m)   =   H
Volume of headspace (L)   = $1000 \times AH$
CH_4 concentration at 0 time (μL L^{-1})   = C_o
CH_4 concentration after time t (μL L^{-1})   = C_t
Change in concentration in time t (μL L^{-1})   = $(C_t - C_o)$
Volume of CH_4 evolved in time t (μL)   = $(C_t - C_o) \times 1000\ AH$
When t is in hours, then flux (mL m^{-2} h^{-1})   = $[(C_t - C_o) \times AH)/(A \times t)]$

Now 22.4 mL of CH_4 is 16 mg at STP

Hence, Flux = $[(C_t - C_o)/t] \times H \times 16/22.4 \times 10000 \times 24$ mg ha^{-1} d^{-1}

Nitrous oxide

The detector used for analysis of N_2O is electron capture detector (ECD), which is used for the detection of those substances which have affinity for electrons. The detector consists of two electrodes, one of which is treated with radioactive ^{63}Ni, which emits beta rays. These high-energy electrons bombard the carrier gas (N_2 or argon mixture) to produce large numbers of low energy (or thermal) secondary electrons. The other positively polarized electrode collects these electrons. This steady state current is reduced when an electrophilic sample component passing through the gap between the two electrodes captures some of these electrons, thus, providing an electrical reproduction of the GC peak. This detector can also contain some other radioactive elements besides ^{63}Ni like tritium or scandium. Although the sensitivity of ^{63}Ni is lower but it remains constant for a longer duration and surpasses the sensitivity of the tritium cell of the same age.

Air samples are analyzed for N_2O concentration using a gas chromatograph equipped with a ^{63}Ni ECD, which is operated at 300-400°C. The temperatures of column, injector and detector are kept at 50°C, 120°C, and 320°C, respectively. Nitrous oxide can be separated from other gaseous components on a Porapak. N column (3m long, stainless steel or nickel with 3.175 mm outside diameter). The flow rates of carrier, back flush and detector purge gases (95% argon + 5% methane or N_2) are kept as 18 $cm^3 min^{-1}$. Gas samples are introduced into a gas sampling loop (size depends upon the sensitivity of the EC detector being used) through an inlet system. Both CO_2 and water vapours are removed from the gas samples. The two absorbent traps are prepared by packing 10-mm millipore syringe filter holders with Ascarite and $MgClO_4$.

A GC-computer interface is used to plot and measure the peak area. N_2O standard (500 ppbV) is used as a primary standard.

Calculation of N_2O flux

Cross-sectional area of the chamber (m^2)	=	A
Headspace (m)	=	H
Volume of headspace (L)	=	$1000 \times AH$
N_2O concentration at 0 time ($\mu L\ L^{-1}$)	=	C_o
N_2O concentration after time t ($\mu L\ L^{-1}$)	=	C_t
Change in concentration in time t ($\mu L\ L^{-1}$)	=	$(C_t - C_o)$
Volume of N_2O evolved in time t (μL)	=	$(C_t - C_o) \times 1000\ AH$
When t is in hours, then flux ($mL\ m^{-2}\ h^{-1}$)	=	$[(C_t - C_o) \times AH]/(A \times t)$

Now 22.4 mL of N_2O is 44 mg at STP

Hence, Flux = $[(C_t - C_o)/t] \times H \times 44/22.4 \times 10000 \times 24$ mg $ha^{-1}\ d^{-1}$

MEASUREMENT TECHNIQUES OF CARBON DIOXIDE EMISSION FROM SOIL

For quantitative analysis of CO_2, two general methods are used in soil respiration research. In the first method, CO_2 that is trapped in an aqueous solution of alkali (usually KOH or NaOH) is precipitated as $BaCO_3$ by the addition of excess $BaCl_2$. The precipitate is collected, washed, dried and weighed. The volumetric analysis for CO_2 trapped in aqueous alkali is a popular method because of its simplicity and high degree of sensitivity. For measurement of CO_2 evolution, alkali of a defined concentration is placed in an open jar above the soil surface, and the area to be measured is covered with a metal cylinder closed at the upper end. The CO_2 evolved from the soil surface is trapped in the cylinder and remains confined there until it is absorbed by the alkali. After a certain period of time, the alkali is removed and its unreacted portion is determined by titration. By subtraction, the amount of CO_2 that combined with the alkali is determined.

Procedure

A CO_2 trap is prepared by pipetting 20 mL of 1N NaOH into a glass jar and placed it on a tripod stand. Immediately the metal cylinder is placed over the alkali trap, and pressed the edge by about 2 cm into the surface of the soil. The cylinder should be shielded from direct sunlight by either covering it with a sheet of wood or a piece of aluminium foil. After exposure of the alkali for 2-4 hours, the jar is removed, covered with lids (airtight seal), and brought to the laboratory for analysis. Controls for this experiment consist of jars of alkali that are incubated in the field in completely sealed metal cylinders by closing the open ends with tightly fitting lids. The airtight seal between lid and cylinder can be obtained by smearing the edge with silicon grease. The alkali solutions from the controls and those exposed to soil air are titrated to determine the quantity of alkali that has not reacted with CO_2. For this purpose, excess $BaCl_2$ is added to the NaOH solution to precipitate the carbonate as insoluble $BaCO_3$. A few drops of phenolphthalein are added as indicator, and titrated with HCl directly in the jar. The acid should be added slowly to avoid contact with and possible dissolution of the precipitated $BaCO_3$. The volume of acid needed to titrate the alkali is noted. The amount of CO_2 evolved from the soil during exposure to alkali may be calculated using the formula:

$$Milligrams\ of\ C\ or\ CO_2 = (B - V)\ NE$$

where, B = volume (mL) of acid needed to titrate NaOH in the jars from the control cylinders, V = volume (mL) of acid needed to titrate the NaOH in the jars exposed to the soil atmosphere, N = normality of the acid, and E = equivalent weight. To express the data in terms of carbon, E = 6; to express it as CO_2, E = 22. Once the milligrams of CO_2-C or CO_2 have been determined, the data are conveniently expressed as mg of CO_2 $m^{-2} h^{-1}$.

MEASURING CARBON DIOXIDE EMISSION BY SOIL RESPIRATOR

The soil respiration, i.e. flux of CO_2 per unit area per unit time, is also measured by placing a closed chamber on the soil and measuring the rate of increase of the CO_2 concentration inside the chamber. The soil respiration system consists of a soil respiration chamber (SRC) and an environmental gas monitor (EGM). For soil respiration, a chamber of known volume is placed on the soil and the rate of increase in CO_2 within the chamber is monitored. With this system, the air is continuously sampled in a closed circuit through the EGM and the soil respiration rate is calculated, displayed and recorded by the analyzer. The air within the chamber is carefully mixed to ensure representative sampling without generating pressure differences, which would affect the evolution of CO_2 from the soil surface.

It is assumed that the rate of increase in CO_2 is linear, though any leakage will cause a decline in its concentration with time. A quadratic equation is fitted to the relationship between the increasing CO_2 concentration and elapsed time.

The soil respiration, i.e. flux of CO_2 per unit area per unit time, is measured by the following equation:

$$R = \frac{(Cn - Co)}{Tn} \times \frac{V}{A}$$

where R is the soil respiration rate (flux of CO_2 per unit area per unit time), Co is the CO_2 concentration at T = 0 and Cn is the concentration at a time Tn, A is the area of soil exposed and V is the total volume of the system.

MEASUREMENT TECHNIQUES OF AMMONIA VOLATILIZATION LOSS FROM SOIL

Several methods have been developed for estimation of ammonia (NH_3) volatilization loss from soil. These include forced draft with externally maintained acid trap, chambers with enclosed acid trap, chambers with acid trap and natural ventilation, mass balance, and micrometeorological techniques. However, the volumetric analysis of NH_3 trapped in aqueous acid is frequently used because of its simplicity and high degree of sensitivity.

Acid trap method

For measurement of NH_3 evolution by this method, acid of a defined concentration is placed in an open jar above the soil surface, and the area to be measured is covered with a metal cylinder that is closed at the upper end. As NH_3 evolves from the soil surface, it is trapped in the cylinder and is confined until the acid absorbs it. After a measured period of time, the acid is removed and the unreacted portion is determined by titration. By sub-traction, the amount of NH_3 that combines with the acid can be determined.

Procedure

A NH_3 trap is prepared by pipetting 20 mL of 1N HCl into a glass jar and placed this onto a tripod. Immediately the metal cylinder is placed over the alkali trap, and the edge is pressed about 2 cm into the surface of the soil. The cylinder should be shielded from direct sunlight by either covering it with a sheet of wood or a piece of aluminum foil. After exposure of the acid for 2-4 hours, the jar is removed, covered them with lids (airtight seal), and brought to the laboratory for analysis. Controls for this experi-ment consist of jars of acid that are incubated in the field in completely sealed metal cylinders by closing the open ends with tightly fitting lids. The airtight seal between lid and cylinder can be obtained by smearing the edge with silicon grease. The acid solutions are titrated from the controls and those exposed to soil air to determine the quantity of acid that has not reacted with NH_3. A few drops of phenolphthalein are added as indicator, and the unreacted HCl is titrated with NaOH directly in the jar. The volume of alkali needed to titrate the acid is noted.

The chambers used for the estimation of CH_4 and N_2O from soil (Figure 1) can also be used for the estimation of NH_3 emission. Filter papers (Whatmann No. 1) soaked in standard sulphuric acid are placed in cham-bers of 50 cm $\times$ 30 cm $\times$ 100 cm made of 6 mm acrylic sheets. The cham-ber is placed on an aluminum channel, inserted 10-cm and the channels are filled with water to make the system air tight. After suitable intervals the filter paper is taken out and titrated against standard NaOH. Another chamber containing filter papers soaked in acid is kept on soil covered with polyethylene sheets, to prevent ammonia coming from soil. This is used to estimate amount of NH_3 present in air inside the chamber. Ammo-nia emission is calculated as the amount of acid neutralized during the pe-riod, the trap is kept inside the chamber. Volatilization loss of N is calcu-lated with the following equation.

Cross sectional area of the chamber (m^2)   =   A
Acid consumed in the chamber kept on polyethylene
covered soil (mL)   = V_o
Acid consumed in the chamber kept in field (mL)   = V_t
Strength of the acid (N)   =   1
Duration of keeping the chamber (h)   =   t

As 1 mL of 1 N acid is equivalent to 0.014 g of NH_3-N, amount of NH_3 evolved (kg ha^{-1} day^{-1}) = $[(V_t - V_o) \times 24 \times 0.014 \times N \times 10]/(t \times A)$

DEVELOPING INVENTORY FOR METHANE AND NITROUS OXIDE EMISSION

There is unreliability in estimation of methane and nitrous oxide emissions from agriculture with its diverse soil, climate, land use types and socio-economic conditions in which it is practiced. What is agriculture's real contribution to greenhouse gas emissions and subsequent climate change can only be answered by preparing a national inventory. This will not only improve estimates of emissions and related impact assessments, but also provide a baseline from which future emission trajectories may be developed to identify and evaluate mitigation strategies.

Methane

Recently, IPCC has outlined a methodology for methane inventory preparation, which takes into account the above parameters (IPCC, 1996). Accordingly the main rice ecosystems are irrigated, rainfed and deepwater. Within each ecosystem are water management systems, which affect the amount of methane emitted during the cropping season.

Emission from rice $(Tg\ yr^{-1}) = \Sigma_i \Sigma j \Sigma_k EF_{ijk} * A_{ijk} * 10^{-12}$

Where i, j and k are categories under which methane emissions from paddy fields vary such as rice ecosystem, water management, cultivar, organic amendment applied, etc.

A_{ijk} = the annual harvested area in m^2 under categories i, j and k.
EF_{ijk} = seasonally integrated emission factor for i, j and k conditions in $g\ m^{-2}$.

The seasonally integrated emission factor is adjusted according to the category is as follows

$EFi = EFc * SFw * SFo * SFs$

where EFi is adjusted seasonally integrated emission factor for a particular harvested area, EFc is seasonally integrated emission factor for continuously flooded fields without organic amendments, SFw is scaling factor to account for differences in ecosystem and water management regime, SFo is scaling factors for different amendment types applied and SFs is scaling factor for soil type.

Nitrous oxide

The emission of N_2O that results from anthropogenic N input occurs through a direct pathway and through a number of indirect pathways including the volatilization losses from synthetic fertilizer and animal manure application, leaching and runoff from applied N to aquatic systems.

The applied N includes synthetic fertilizer, animal manure and also the sewage sludge applied to soils. The volatilization of applied N as ammonia (NH_3) and oxides of nitrogen (NO_x) is followed by deposition as ammonium (NH_4) and oxides of nitrogen (NO_x) on soils and water and accounts for indirect nitrous oxide emissions from soils. Thus, the emission of N_2O has been calculated in two steps: a) direct N_2O emission from agricultural soils and b) indirect N_2O emission from agricultural soils.

Direct N_2O Emission

$$N_2O_{direct}-N = \{(F_{SN} + F_{AM} + F_{BN} + F_{CR}) * EF_1\} + (F_{OS} * EF_2)$$

where, F_{SN} denotes the annual amount of synthetic fertilizer N applied to soil adjusted to account for the amount that volatilizes as NH_3 and NO_x.

$$F_{SN} = N_{FERT} * (1 - Frac_{GASF})$$

where, N_{FERT} denotes the total amount of synthetic fertilizer consumed annually. $Frac_{GASF}$ is the fraction of fertilizer that volatilizes as NH_3 and NO_x (IPCC, 1996). Extents of volatilization depend on several of soil, plant and climatic factors. Amount of N applied, soil pH, temperature and soil moisture are the major factors affecting volatilization loss of N. F_{AM} denotes the annual amount of animal manure nitrogen intentionally applied to soils adjusted to account for volatilization as NH_3 and NO_x.

$$F_{AM} = \sum_T (N_{(T)} * N_{ex\,(T)}) * (1 - Frac_{GASM}) [1 - (Frac_{FUEL} + Frac_{PRP} + Frac_{COLLEC} + Frac_{FEED} + Frac_{CONST})]$$

where, T stands for each defined livestock category/species. In this calculation three categories of livestock that are bovine, sheep and goat have been taken. N_T is the number of animals in each category. $N_{ex(T)}$ is the annual average nitrogen excretion rate per head for each livestock category.

$Frac_{GASM}$ is the fraction of N that volatilizes as NH_3 & NO_x, which is 15% of the N content of manure. $Frac_{FUEL}$ denotes animal manure that is burned for fuel. $Frac_{PRP}$ is the fraction of animal manure that is deposited on to soil by grazing livestock. $Frac_{CONST}$ is the fraction of animal manure that is used as construction. $Frac_{FEED}$ is the fraction of animal manure that is being used as feed. This fraction has been assumed to be zero in present estimation. $Frac_{COLLEC}$ is the loss during collection of dung.

F_{BN} stands for the amount of N fixed by N-fixing crops cultivated annually.

$$F_{BN} = Crop_{BF} * Frac_{NCRBF}$$

where $Crop_{BF}$ is seed yield of N-fixing crops. $Frac_{NCRBF}$ is the fraction of crop biomass that is nitrogen.

F_{CR} is the amount of N in crop residue returned to soil annually, which is calculated using the following relationship.

$$F_{CR} = (Crop_{ST} * Frac_{NCRST} + Crop_{SBF} * Frac_{NCRSBF})$$

where, $Crop_{ST}$ is the amount of straw of non-N fixing crops incorporated to the soil as residue. $Crop_{SBF}$ is the amount of straw of N fixing crops incorporated to the soil as residue that can be calculated by the following formula.

$$Straw\ Yield = (Grain\ Yield/Harvest\ Index)-Grain\ Yield.$$

$Frac_{NCRST}$ is the nitrogen content of residue of non-N fixing crops and $Frac_{NCRSBF}$ is the N content of residue of N fixing crops.
F_{OS} is the area of organic soils harvested (area of organic soils cultivated annually).
EF_1 is the emission factor for N_2O-N emitted from the various nitrogen additions to the soil.
EF_2 is the emission factor for N_2O emitted from cultivation of organic soils.

Indirect N_2O Emission

$$N_2O_{indirect} = N_2O_{(G)} + N_2O_{(L)}$$

where, $N_2O_{indirect}$ denotes the emission of N_2O-N indirectly from agriculture.
$N_2O_{(G)}$ is the N_2O produced from volatilization of applied synthetic fertilizer and animal manure N and its subsequent atmospheric deposition as NO_x and NH_4.

$$N_2O_{(G)} = [(N_{FERT} * Frac_{GASF}) + (\Sigma_T(N_{(T)} * Nex_{(T)} * Frac_{GASM})] * EF_4$$

where, N_{FERT} is the amount of synthetic fertilizer consumed annually. $Frac_{GASF}$ is the fraction of fertilizer that volatilizes as NH_3 and NO_x. $\Sigma_T(N_{(T)} * Nex_{(T)}$ denotes the amount of animal manure nitrogen excreted annually. T is each defined livestock category. N_T is the number of animals in each category. $N_{ex(T)}$ is the annual nitrogen excretion rate per head for each livestock category.
$Frac_{GASM}$ is the fraction of manure that volatilizes as NH_3 & NO_x.
EF_4 is the emission factor for N_2O emissions from atmospheric NH_3 and NO_x.

Deposited N from leaching and runoff

$$N_2O_{(L)} = N_{FERT} + \{ \Sigma_T(N_{(T)} * Nex_{(T)} * [1-(Frac_{FUEL-AM} + Frac_{PRP-AM} + Frac_{COLLEC} + Frac_{FEED-AM} + Frac_{CNST-M})]\} * Frac_{LEACH} * EF_5$$

where, $N_2O_{(L)}$ is N_2O produced from leaching and runoff of applied fertilizer and animal manure N, $Frac_{FUEL-AM}$ denotes animal manure that is burned for fuel, $Frac_{PRP-AM}$ is the fraction of animal manure that is deposited on to soil by grazing livestock. $Frac_{COLLEC}$ is the loss of dung during collection. $Frac_{CONST-AM}$ is the fraction of animal manure that is used as construction, $Frac_{FEED-AM}$ is the fraction of animal manure that is being fed, $Frac_{LEACH}$ is the fraction of N lost through leaching, and EF_5 is the emission factor for deposited N from leaching and run-off (kg N_2O- N kg^{-1} N leached and runoff).

Total N_2O-N emission:

$$N_2O\text{-}N_{TOTAL} = N_2O\text{-}N_{DIRECT} + N_2O\text{-}N_{INDIRECT}$$

LIST OF ABBREVIATIONS

F_{SN}	Amount of fertilizer N applied to soil adjusted for gas loss
N_{FERT}	Amount of fertilizer consumed annually
$Frac_{GASF}$	Fraction of fertilizer that volatilizes as NH_3 and NO_x
F_{AM}	Amount of animal manure nitrogen applied to soil adjusted for gas loss
T	Each defined livestock category/species
N_T	Number of animals in each category
$N_{ex(T)}$	Average nitrogen excretion rate per head for each livestock category
$Frac_{GASM}$	Fraction of N that volatilizes as NH_3 & NO_x from manure
$Frac_{FUEL}$	Fraction of animal manure that is burned for fuel
$Frac_{PRP}$	Fraction of animal manure that is deposited by grazing livestock
$Frac_{CONST}$	Fraction of animal manure that is used as construction
$Frac_{FEED}$	Fraction of animal manure that is being used as feed
F_{BN}	Amount of N fixed by N-fixing crops
$Crop_{BF}$	Seed yield of N-fixing crops
$Frac_{NCRBF}$	Nitrogen content of crop biomass
F_{CR}	Amount of N in crop residue returned to soil annually
$Crop_{ST}$	Amount of straw of non-N fixing crops incorporated as residue
$Crop_{SBF}$	Amount of straw of N fixing crops incorporated as residue
$Frac_{NCRST}$	Nitrogen content of residue of N fixing crops
$Frac_{NCRSBF}$	N content of residue of N fixing crops
F_{OS}	Area of organic soils harvested
EF_1	Emission factor for N_2O-N emitted from the nitrogen addition to soil
EF_2	Emission factor for N_2O emitted from cultivation of organic soils
$N_2O_{(G)}$	N_2O produced from volatilization of applied synthetic fertilizer and animal manure N and its subsequent atmosphere deposition as NO_x and NH_4.

CHAPTER 7

Global warming and soil microbial activity

ANITA CHAUDHARY, S. PURI, N. KALRA *and* H. PATHAK

"The world gets better everyday – then worse again in the evening."—Kin Hubbard

ATMOSPHERIC COMPOSITION IS KEPT at a close homeostasis by the activity of biosphere that is largely dominated by various microbial processes, resulting in the biogeochemical cycling of essential elements both within the ecosystems and on a global basis. These cycles highly affect the environment of the planet. Paleo-climatic evidences suggest that the evolution of photosynthetic oxygen by cyanobacteria led to a shift from a highly reduced anoxic to an oxic atmosphere, paving the way for evolution of higher forms of life. These cycles have remained almost stable for millions of years. The tiny miniscule components of the ecosystem, i.e. microbes have largely been responsible for the sustainability of these stable conditions. However, recent phenomenon of global warming and possible climate change may perturb the stability of the ecosystem and have more pronounced effects on the microbial communities, the critical component of the ecosystem.

Soil is a favourable habitat for microorganisms as it provides shelter and nutrition to the microbes. In return, microorganisms contribute immensely in determining soil fertility through humus formation, cycling of nutrients, and soil aggregation. Microbial processes are responsible for the degradation and formation of organic matter and the temperature at which these processes occur and easy availability of substrates are likely to control the rate of organic mater transformation, provided other soil conditions such as moisture, pH, oxygen supply and clay content do not vary. Soil is the most dominant component in the cycling of greenhouse gases because of the high abundance and diversity of microbes in it. They act as source as well as sink for these gases (Table 1). In this chapter we shall discuss (i) the role of microbes in production and consumption of greenhouse gases, and (ii) impact of global warming on soil microbial activity.

Table 1: Importance of microbes as sources of greenhouse gases (Modified from Conard, 1995)

Green-house gases	Relative importance as source			Microorganism invloved	Relation to oxygen
	Microbe	Animal/Plant	Human		
Carbon di oxide	86	10	4	Autotroph (-)¶	Oxic
				Heterotroph (+)	Oxic
Methane	26	17	57	Methanotrophs (-)	Oxic
				Nitrifiers (-)	Oxic
Nitrous oxide	50	—	50	Methanogens (+)	Anoxic
				Nitrifiers (+)	Oxic
				Denitrifiers (+)	Anoxic

¶ (+) and (-) indicate processes leading to production and consumption of greenhouse gases, respectively

MICROORGANISMS IN PRODUCTION AND CONSUMPTION OF GREENHOUSE GASES

Carbon dioxide in the atmosphere represents the most actively recycled reservoir of carbon by virtue of the process of photosynthesis and respiration. The fixed organic matter is recycled as CO_2 to the atmosphere and new cell mass in the soil by the catabolic activities of heterotrophs during aerobic respiration.

Formation of methane, i.e. methanogenesis, is predominantly a microbial process carried out under anaerobic conditions by a specific group of autotrophs, i.e. obligate anaerobic archae-bacteria, e.g. *Methanobacterium* sp., *Synthrophomonas* sp. with the utilization of CO_2/H_2 as substrates. Heterotrophic genesis of methane is carried out by the growth of heterotrophs on formate, acetate and methanol, produced by other microbes of the community that normally develop during anaerobiosis. In upland soils, where oxic conditions are prevalent, a group of chemoautotrophic, obligate aerobes called methanotrophs, e.g. *Methylococccus capsulatus*, consume methane. There are culturable and nonculturable methanotrophs. The former group has a low affinity for CH_4 and, therefore, metabolize it only at a higher concentration. Normally these bacteria are present as cysts or exospores and become active only in the presence of sufficiently high concentration of methane. The later group defined as non-culturable has a high affinity for methane and is able to metabolize it even at the current atmospheric CH_4 concentration (1.7 ppmV). Besides the methanotrophs, nitrifying bacteria also carry out methane oxidation and exhibit a high affinity for CH_4, similar to that of uncultivable CH_4 oxidizing methanotrpophs.

Nitrous Oxide is produced in the soil environment as an intermediate in nitrification and denitrification processes in the nitrogen cycle. Production of N_2O from nitrification, carried out by ammonium oxidizers like *Nitrosomonas europaea, Nitrospira briensis, Nitrosolobus multiformis, Nitrococcus mobilis* and *Nitrosovibrio tenuis* and nitrite oxidizers like *Nitrobacter winogradskyi* and *Nitrobacter vulgaris* is favoured in aerated moist soils. The denitrification process, carried out by denitrifiers (*Pseudomonas* and *Alcaligenes*), occurs in anaerobic soil conditions. The processes involved in the N_2O consumption have not yet been studied in detail because the uptake of N_2O by soil from atmosphere has only been observed occasionally. Still, some evidence points towards the involvement of denitrifiers in its consumption under anaerobic conditions. Another microbial process contributing towards its removal is the dissimilatory reduction of nitrate to ammonia by anaerobic bacteria, e.g. *Wollinella succinogenes*, through the process of anaerobic respiration (Teraguchi and Hollocher, 1989).

EFFECT OF GLOBAL WARMING ON MICROBIAL ACTIVITY

Global warming manifested through increased temperature and atmospheric carbon dioxide concentration is likely to cause direct as well as indirect effects on the microbial community.

Effect of increased atmospheric CO_2 concentration

Effect of increase in CO_2 concentration in the atmosphere will have indirect rather than any direct effect on soil-microbial community because the concentration of CO_2 in soil is 10-50 times higher than that in the atmosphere. Effect of increase in CO_2 concentration on plant growth would be reflected in a higher rate of photosynthesis, leading to more plant growth. Consequently, there will be greater rhizodeposition and higher rate of microbial biomass production. Since the rate of rhizodeposition may not be proportional to the rate of increase in microbial population, a time may come, when the demand for substrates would exceed the supply and the microorganisms would use the existing pool of soil organic matter (SOM), resulting in higher mineralization. The byproducts of this reaction will further enhance the growth of plants, setting in a vicious cycle (Figure 1). Although there would be a simultaneous regeneration of SOM pool via addition of carbon in the form of plant litter, but increased C:N in plant tissues

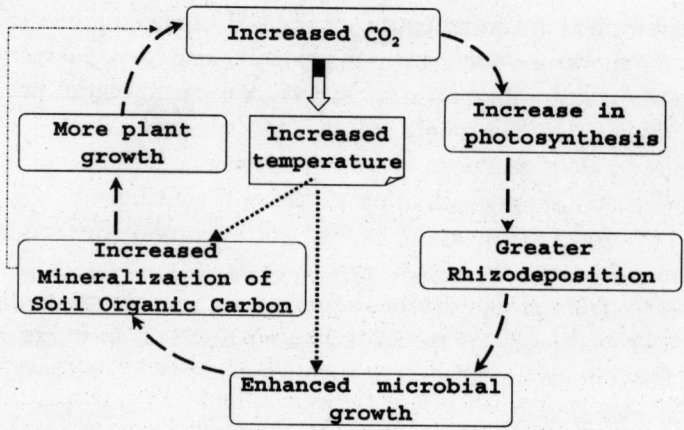

Figure 1: Cascading effect of the dynamics of carbon dioxide on soil fertility

growing actively under such conditions may result in recalcitrant organic matter because of high concentrations of phenolic compounds (Gorissen *et al.*, 1995). Thus, there may be a net deprivation of soil organic carbon pool. Consequently, CO_2-induced changes may generate intra- and inter-specific competition between microbes for scarce nutrients and habitats leading to shifts in microbial community. With the increase in CO_2 concentration, there may be slow changes in the evolutionary pattern of the microbes, as has been observed during the evolutionary period of earth.

Effect of increase in temperature

The most prominent effect of increase in temperature would be the enhanced growth rate of microbes, resulting in an increase in the rate of decomposition of SOM. Temperature responses of biological systems are expressed as a Q_{10} function, i.e. relative change in rate with a 10°C rise in temperature.

$$Q_{10} = (k_2/k_1)^{[10(T2-T1)]}$$

where, k_2 and k_1 are the rate constants for a process of interest at two observed temperatures, T2 and T1. For example, a Q_{10} of 2 means that the rate of a particular process at 20°C would be twice as fast as that at 10°C.

In general, the processes of production (photosynthetic rates) and decomposition (respiration) respond differently towards changes in temperatures. Rates of respiration increase exponentially with temperature with no upper limit, whereas, photosynthesis increases linearly and shows saturation at higher temperature. The kinetics of these processes underly the concern that global warming could trigger a net release of CO_2 from soils to atmosphere, leading to a positive feedback to global warming.

It is widely known that certain groups of microorganisms are well adapted to particular temperature regimes. Temperature can illicit changes in microbial community composition, which manifests itself in the propagation of dominant populations at higher temperatures having the ability to metabolize substrates that are not used by members of microbial community at lower temperatures. Altered microbial community structures can be depicted by the changes in the phospholipid fatty acid profiles (PLFA) of the communities (Zogg *et al.*, 1997). Phospholipids are membrane components of living cell and make up a relatively constant proportion of the biomass of an organism. In general, PLFA profiles show decreasing unsaturation, greater chain length and larger number of cyclopropyl fatty acids at higher temperatures.

Interplay of CO_2, temperature, nitrogen availability and other factors

Concentration of CO_2 and temperature as independent variables will cause inconsistent changes in the soil organic matter composition and quality, as discussed above, but in reality it is the interaction of these two variables that will determine the quantum of soil CO_2 effluxes in different regions. Moreover, these factors again will not act independently, but in conjunction with certain other factors such as nitrogen availability, moisture, substrate quality, etc. Increased belowground carbon allocation in the form of rhizodeposits could cause soils to act as sinks for C at elevated CO_2 concentrations in as far as soil C is limited by inputs rather than by its C-protection capacity (i.e. the maximum amount of carbon that can be associated with clay and silt particles in soil). Not only the amount of carbon deposited in the soil but also the output through decomposition may be affected by the CO_2 due to changes in the substrate quality or microbial activity. Soil microorganisms will preferentially use the rhizodeposits because they are more easily decomposable, provided that sufficient N is available. Actually increased microbial biomass might cause higher denitrification rates, immobilize more soil N and thus initiate a shortage of N for the plants. Also, an increased decomposition of C into more resilient molecules would mean an increased immobilization of soil N. At low N microorganisms would have to utilize soil organic matter as main substrate, again suggesting a means for loss of SOM.

Moisture is another critical factor for determination of the effect of climate change on CH_4 consumption and CO_2 production. Under warmer but drier conditions in some wetlands, CH_4 consumption rather than production would be enhanced as water table levels would drop and the depth of aerated soil would increase (Whalen and Reeburgh, 1990). Whereas, in uplands, drying could suppress CH_4 consumption due to water stress on soil microbes. In drier conditions, respiration and CO_2 production would decrease and will show an increase under wetter conditions.

Effects of climate change would be region-specific. In tropical regions, high temperatures and humidity promote rapid decomposition and leaching, and the result is a greater proportion of nutrient – poor, highly weathered soils that are more susceptible to losses of soil organic matter. Nitrification is accelerated in warmer soils, if they are well-aerated and denitrification also increases with temperature, whereas high temperatures inhibit microbial nitrogen fixation. Tropical regions with smaller soil C reserves and lower anticipated warming could be of lesser significance, but variations in sensitivities of photosynthesis and respiration processes to temperature, as discussed earlier, suggest a potential efflux of CO_2. Production processes like photosynthesis is less sensitive to changes in temperature than microbial respiration (and decomposition rates) at higher temperatures such as those existing in the tropics. This is because the process of photosynthesis is already operating in its saturation range as far as increase in temperature is concerned. However, rates of soil respiration will increase exponentially with temperature, causing a greater absolute effect on CO_2 efflux in a warmer region, compared to cooler one.

Temperate regions with larger stocks of soil C, coupled with greater predicted warming, could also lead to massive efflux of CO_2, but the pattern would not be a rapid one, as in the tropics. The less rate of organic matter turnover and a greater response of net primary productivity towards temperature changes at low temperatures, may lead to short-term carbon storage in this region. This is further evidenced by the presence of complexed organic matter reserves in these areas. With increasing temperatures, the photosynthetic rates will increase linearly as the process is not yet operating in the saturation range whereas decomposition would not increase to a large extent initially because of its lesser sensitivity to increase in temperature at lower temperature ranges. But, if we take a long-term scenario for the temperate regions wherein we consider continuous increase in temperature due to global warming, these regions would represent a more robust and sustainable potential for CO_2 emissions. This may be due to the temperature increases to a large extent over a period of time, which will result in a shift in the temperature sensitivity of decomposition/respiration processes from low to high. This would eventually lead to an exponential increase in the decomposition in these regions too, like the tropics and since these regions have an almost untouched and huge organic carbon stock, this would lead to a much more sustained carbon loss in terms of CO_2 emissions over a period of 100 years or more. Thus, losses of soil organic matter are evident in the temperate as well as the tropics, but the pattern would be of a more immediate and rapid type in the tropics, spanning a few decades, whereas in the temperate regions, it would be of a slower but more sustained type, occurring over a longer period of time.

BIOTECHNOLOGICAL APPROACHES FOR THE MITIGATION OF GREENHOUSE GAS EMISSION

Depending on the agro-climatic zone of a region and the predicted extent of global warming in that region, vegetation of the area can be planned. Microbial population of the region can also be altered. For example, if N limitation is expected in soil, legumes can be grown to fix more atmospheric N. Also, mass inoculums of organism that act as the sinks for the prominent greenhouse gas can be released in the soils or substances promoting their growth can be added. Release of unculturable populations of CH_4 consumers or promoting their populations will be an option to reduce CH_4 emission. Sea planktons, the major chunk of the autotrophic populations can be considered as a potential sink for CO_2. Special efforts have to be undertaken to promote their extensive growth by addition of limiting nutrients, specially Fe to the water bodies. The efficiency of these microbes could be enhanced by the use of bio-technological tools.

CHAPTER 8

Impact of climate change on Indian agriculture

A. CHATTERJEE, H. PATHAK, U.A. SONI *and* N. KALRA

"We can only change the world by changing men."
—Charles Wells

CONTINUOUS BUILD UP OF greenhouse gasses in the atmosphere is causing global warming. This in turn may change the global climate, which would impact local agriculture, and therefore, influence the world's food supply. Changes in the temperature, solar radiation, and precipitation may affect the productivity of various agro-ecological systems. Climate change will also have an economic impact including changes in farm profitability, prices, supply and demand and could have far-reaching effects on the patterns of trade among the nations. Though there has been significant advancement of knowledge in understanding and predicting the important facets of climatic variability as well as crops and farming systems in the recent past, uncertainties in global climatic scenario and projections limit the prediction of climatic impact on agriculture. Both the positive and negative effects of climate change on agriculture have been projected depending on the crop, inputs and agro-climatic region (Baker and Allen, 1993).

The topographic and geographic location of India, which influence the climate of the region, not only have a great variety of natural resources, including surface and ground water availability, forestry and vegetation but also have a very rich collection of flora and fauna. Changes to the present climate system may affect a wide variety of eco-systems and socio-economic sectors in the country with corresponding impacts on water resources, agriculture, forestry and other sectors. The mean temperature in India is projected to increase by 0.1°C to 0.3°C in kharif and 0.3°C to 0.7°C in rabi by 2010 and to 0.4°C to 2.0°C in kharif and 1.1°C to 4.5°C in rabi by 2070 (IPCC, 1996). Mean rainfall is projected to change by ±10% by 2070. At the same time there is an increased possibility of climate extremes such as the timing of onset of monsoon, intensities and frequencies of droughts and floods.

IMPACT OF CLIMATE CHANGE ON CROP PRODUCTIVITY

As yields in some of the most productive regions of the world are approaching a plateau or even declining (Pathak *et al.*, 2003a), the likely effect of climate change on crop production adds to the already complex problem. On one hand, an increase in the CO_2 level in the atmosphere would increase crop yield mainly by stimulating photosynthetic processes and improving water use efficiency. On the other hand, the effect of increased temperature would largely be negative because of increased respiration and a shortened vegetative and grain-filling period. The net effect of an increase in CO_2 and temperature is complicated and depends on the relative effects of both variables in a given region. The direct effects of climatic change on crops include effects on photosynthesis, respiration, phenology and yield attributing characters. The indirect effects include shift in climate and agricultural zones; effects on soil organic matter, soil erosion, soil water availability, soil salinization and alkalinization; desertification; and pests and diseases. The possible impact of climate change on the productivity of major crops in India are dealt with in the following section.

Wheat

Wheat is an important cereal crop, grown from 15°N to 32°N; 72°E to 92°E, sea level to fairly high altitudes and experiences different temperatures during the crop season. These climatic differences associated with the location together with the annual variation in climatic parameters strongly affect the growth and productivity of wheat. Simulated potential and irrigated wheat yields have latitudinal dependence arising due to variations in climatic and soil characteristics. It has been estimated that an increase of 1°C temperature coupled with carbon-dioxide concentration change to 425 ppm would have no effect or slightly increase the productivity in irrigated as well as rainfed environments, particularly in northern India. Increase in temperature by 2°C will reduce the potential yields but will have small effects on the irrigated yield in northern India. On the other hand the effect of climatic change will be more pronounced in the central India where the potential yield is already low. In sub-tropical (above 23°N) regions there would be a small decrease in potential yields (1.5-5.8%) but in tropical regions the decrease would be 17-18 % (Aggarwal and Kalra, 1994).

Thereby the beneficial effect of increase in CO_2 in north India, however, is nullified by increase in temperature (1.5 to 3.3°C). It could be concluded that in a climate change scenario irrigated wheat productivity is likely to suffer more in eastern and central India compared to northern regions of the country (Aggarwal *et al.*, 1998).

Rice

Rice is another important crop in the world with about 525 million tonnes being produced from about 148 million hectares (IRRI, 2000). It is grown over a considerable geographical range from 45°N to 40°S, elevations more than 2500 m above mean sea level with the average daily temperature in the range of 20 to 30°C.

The overall effect of an increase in CO_2 and temperature is more complicated due to the variety of cropping systems and technology used. A temperature increase at higher latitudes generally decreases yields by reducing the crop duration. In the central region of unstable and uncertain agriculture, rice productivity is low due to increasing trend in the instability i.e. extreme fluctuations of rainfall. In the eastern region, long duration varieties would suffer more from water stress conditions as compared to medium and short duration varieties during the reproductive and maturity stages.

An increase of rice yield to the tune of 12% with the projected climate change scenario (increase of temperature by 1.5°C and rainfall ↓↑ by 2 mm at a CO_2 concentration of 460 ppm) in southern India was estimated by Saseendran *et al.* (1999). But reductions in anthesis period and crop maturity period, caused by the increase in temperature in the event of climate change, will lead to reductions in yields.

Maize

Being a plant with C_4 photosynthetic pathway the gain in productivity due to increase in the atmospheric CO_2 level is generally lower than the C_3 pathway-plants. On the other hand increase in temperature would decrease the yield from the present day condition for Indian environments (Chatterjee, 1998). The beneficial effect of 700-ppm CO_2 would be nullified by an increase of only 0.9°C in temperature. Further increase in temperature would always result in lowering the yields irrespective of the increase in CO_2.

Sugarcane

Sugarcane is one of the most important cash crops of the country and plays a pivotal role in country's agricultural and industrial economy. An adverse effect of rise in temperature on cane yield would be more pronounced in moderate to limited water supply situations. For every 1°C rise in temperature, there would be a significant reduction of yield of this crop. But rise in CO_2 concentration could compensate the negative effects of temperature rise (Chattopadhyay, 2000).

Brassica

With the increases in temperature and atmospheric CO_2 concentration, production of *Brassica* is likely to increase and to be shifted to relatively drier regions where it is not being grown at present.

IMPACT OF CLIMATE CHANGE ON SOIL

The soil system responds to the short-term events such as episodic infiltration of rainfall and also undergoes long-term changes such as physical and chemical weathering due to climatic change. The potential changes in the soil forming factors directly resulting from global climatic change would be in the organic matter supply, temperature regimes, hydrology and changes in the potential evapotranspiration. The most rapid process of chemical or mineralogical change under changing external conditions would be an increase in the salt concentration. As the extent of saline-sodic soils in India is already high, further increase in salinity areas will have a far-reaching effect on food production. The distribution of land resources and soil productivity will change from the present pattern on account of

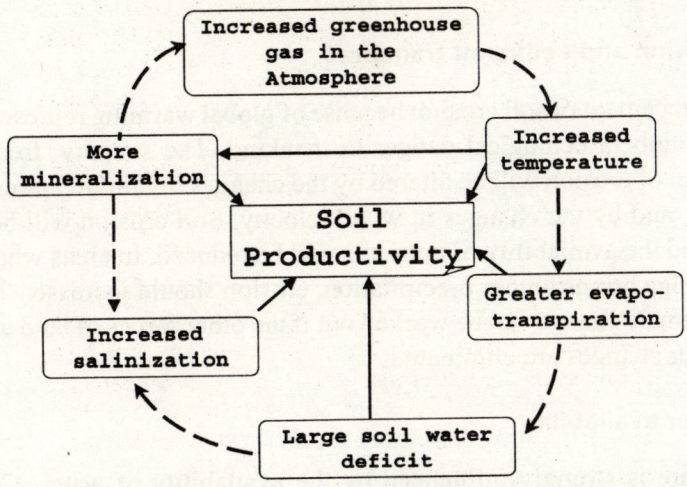

Figure 1: Impact on soild productivity due to global warming

not only sea level rise but also due to high temperature and high PET as schematized in Figure 1.

Soil organic matter content and fertility

Chemical reactions that affect soil minerals and organic matter are strongly influenced by higher soil and water temperature. The most important process likely to be affected by the climatic change, particularly increased temperature, is the accelerated decomposition of organic matter, which releases the nutrients in short-run but may reduce the fertility on long term basis. Soil temperature also affects the rates of nutrient uptake. Both the organic matter and C:N will diminish in the warmer conditions as a result of accelerated decomposition by the microbial action, where clay content tends to increase due to the accelerated weathering of primary minerals. If we assume that the CO_2 fertilization effects cause the yields to increase in some locations, more nutrients will be removed from the soil at each harvest. Nitrogen is made available to plants in a biologically usable form through the action of bacteria in the soil. Nitrification is inhibited in cooler regions and accelerated in warmer regions if they are well aerated. Denitrification also increases with soil temperature. The rate of P uptake too is enhanced as soil temperature rises. However, high soil temperature may have a depressing effect on the symbiotic nitrogen-fixing bacteria. This process of nitrogen fixation, associated with the greater root development, is also predicted to increase in the warmer conditions and with higher CO_2, if soil moisture is not limiting. Drier soil conditions will suppress both root growth and decomposition of organic matter and will increase vulnerability to erosion.

Soil erosion and sediment transport

The enhancement of soil erosion because of global warming represents the most incumbent ecological danger to mankind. The severity, frequency and extent of erosion will be altered by the changes in rainfall amount and intensity, and by the changes in wind velocity. Soil erosion will become severe and the availability of nutrients will be reduced. In areas where climate change brings higher precipitation, erosion should increase. The effect of climate change can be worked out if the other forces of land use and land cover changes are eliminated.

Soil water availability

Agriculture is strongly influenced by the availability of water. Climate change will modify the rainfall, evaporation, runoff and soil moisture storage. The occurrence of moisture stress during flowering, pollination, and grain filling is harmful to most crops and particularly so to corn, soyabean, and wheat. Increased evaporation from the soil and accelerated transpiration from the plants will cause moisture stress, as a result, there will be a need to develop the crop varieties of greater drought tolerance. The impact of climate change on water availability needs to be established on watershed or command area basis where other driving factors are also taken into consideration.

DESERTIFICATION

Desertification, a cause for the land degradation, and soil loss, threatens over one third of the world's total land surface. Any change in climate which results in expansion or contraction of arid, semi arid and sub humid areas will alter the extent of the area in which desertification is considered to be occurring. The global climate change may in turn accelerate desertification, if higher temperature increases the evaporation or if rainfall decreases.

PESTS, DISEASES AND WEEDS

Pest, disease and weed are early indicators of climate change as it will potentially alter the pest/weed—host relationship by affecting (i) pest/weed population, (ii) host population and (iii) pest/weed—host interactions. The temperature patterns, rainfall or humidity and season length, all have an effect on the development and distribution of pest and diseases. Climate change is likely to cause a spread of tropical and subtropical species into temperate areas and to increase the numbers of many temperate species currently limited by the low temperature at high latitudes. An increase in temperature will lead to more opportunity for the population growth in areas already affected by the pest. Incidence of pest and diseases would be most severe in tropical regions due to favorable climate/weather conditions, multiple cropping and availability of alternate pests throughout the year.

IMPACT OF CLIMATE CHANGE ON AGRICULTURAL LANDS AND ZONES

Global climate change also has the potential to alter the geographical distribution of agricultural lands as well as the absolute amount of land, which can be cultivated. As temperature increases, climatic zones can be expected to shift and some areas may be rendered unfit for food production. Some lands, which are presently uncultivable due to climatic factors, may become suitable, while on the other side, currently arable areas may become unproductive. In South and Southeast Asia, it means that agriculture will tend to migrate northward. Increased temperatures can also be expected to raise the altitudinal limits of cultivation. Agriculture may be able to expand to higher elevations. If this occurs, however, agriculture may come into conflict with high-altitude livestock pastures. There is also the danger that agriculture may encroach upon natural habitats. In any case, the social adjustments necessitated by such shifts in agricultural zones will be immense.

TECHNOLOGICAL POTENTIAL OF INDIAN AGRICULTURE TO ADAPT IN THE CHANGING CLIMATE

Change in agricultural technologies offer good promise for adapting to climate change. Some of the important ones are:

In case of short-season crops such as wheat, rice, barley, oats, and many vegetable crops, extension of the growing season may allow more crops in a year. However, for the subtropical and tropical areas where growing season is limited by precipitation or where the cropping intensity is already higher, the ability to extend the growing season may be more limited and depends on the changes in the precipitation pattern.

For major crops, varieties exist with a wide range of maturities and climatic tolerances. Longer-season cultivars were shown to provide a steadier yield under more variable conditions. In general, such changes may lead to higher yields or may only partly offset losses in yields or profitability. Crop diversification in Canada (Cohen *et al.,* 1992) and in China (Hulme *et al.,* 1992) has been identified as an adaptive response. Moreover, the genetic base is broad for most crops but limited for some (e.g., kiwi fruit). Heat, drought and pest resistance, salt tolerance, and general improvements in crop yield and quality would be beneficial. Genetic engineering and gene mapping offer the potential for introducing a wider range of traits.

Climate change will also affect future water supplies. Water and nutrient management has to be redefined in various agro-ecologies to meet the climate change. Irrigated agriculture, is in general, less negatively affected than dryland agriculture but adding irrigation is costly and subject to the availability of water supplies. There is wide scope for enhancing irrigation efficiency through adoption of drip irrigation systems and other water-conserving technologies but successful adoption will require substantial changes in management of irrigation systems and the pricing of water. Competition for water is likely to increase, necessitating changes in the management and pricing of water regardless of whether and how climate changes.

Added nitrogen and other fertilizers would likely be necessary to take full advantage of the increase in CO_2 level in the atmosphere but may have deleterious effects on humans and aquatic ecosystems.

Minimum and reduced tillage technologies in combination with planting of cover crops and green manure crops offer substantial possibilities to reverse existing soil organic matter, soil erosion, and nutrient loss and to combat potential further losses due to climate change.

Linking agricultural management to seasonal climate predictions (currently largely based on the El Niño Southern Oscillation phenomenon), where such predictions can be made with reliability, can allow management to adapt incrementally to climate change. Management/climate predictor links are an important and growing part of agricultural extension in both developed and developing countries.

Adoption of new or different technologies depends on many factors: economic incentives; varying resource and climatic conditions; the existence of other technologies (transportation systems and markets); the availability of information; and the remaining economic life of equipment and structures (such as dams and water supply systems).

Specific technologies can only provide a successful adaptive response if they are adopted in appropriate situations. A variety of issues need to be considered, including land-use planning, watershed management, disaster vulnerability assessment, consideration of port and rail adequacy, trade policy, and the various programmes that the countries use to encourage or control production, limit food prices, and manage resource inputs to agriculture.

Existing gaps between best yields and the average farm yields remain unexplained but many are due in part to socio-economic reasons; which adds considerable uncertainty to estimates of the potential for adaptation particularly in developing countries. Yield gap analysis to analyze the factors responsible has to be linked with climate change and variability in order to design the techniques to reduce the yield gap. Important strategies for improving the ability of agriculture to respond to diverse demands and pressures, drawn from past efforts to transfer technology and provide assistance for agricultural development, include:

- Improved training and general education of populations dependent on agriculture, particularly in India where education of rural workers is currently limited. Agronomic experts can provide guidance on possible strategies and technologies that may be effective. Farmers must evaluate and compare these options to find those appropriate to their needs and the circumstances of their farm.
- Identification of the present vulnerabilities of agricultural systems,

causes of resource degradation, and existing systems that are resilient and sustainable. Strategies that are effective in dealing with current climate variability and resource degradation are also likely to increase resilience and adaptability to future climate change.

- Agricultural research centers and experiment stations can examine the 'robustness' of present farming systems (i.e. their resilience to extremes of heat, cold, frost, water shortage, pest damage and other factors) and also test the robustness of new farming strategies as they are developed to meet changes in climate, technology, prices, costs and other factors.
- Interactive communication that brings research results to farmers and farmers' problems, perspectives and successes to researchers is an essential part of the agricultural research system.
- Agricultural research provides a foundation for adaptation. Genetic variability for most major crops is wide relative to projected climate change. Preservation and effective use of this genetic material would provide the basis for new variety development. Continually changing climate is likely to increase the value of networks of experiment stations that can share genetic material and research results.
- Food programmes and other social security programmes would provide insurance against local supply changes.
- Infrastructure facilities like transportation, distribution and market need to be improved.
- Existing policies may limit efficient response to climate change. Changes in policies such as crop subsidy schemes, land tenure systems, water pricing and allocation, and international trade barriers could increase the adaptive capability of agriculture.

Many of the above strategies will be beneficial regardless of how or whether climate changes. Building the capability to detect change and evaluate possible responses is fundamental to successful adaptation. Thus, even without having clear predictions of climate change, it is possible to identify some strategies that reduce potential vulnerability.

There is fair degree of agreement that continuing build up of heat absorbing gases in the atmosphere is causing global climate change. Climatic changes expected to occur in the near future are already showing their impact. This will influence the global climatic patterns and hence modify the crop productivity. Global climate change is definitely going to affect major crops like rice, wheat, maize, sugarcane and *Brassica*, in India. Various locations in India will be affected differently under climate change, with some locations gaining (rice in Southern India and *Brassica* in Northern

India) in agriculture productivity while others losing (wheat, sugarcane, maize in Northern India). Climate is the least manageable of all resources, hence to avert the ill effects of climate change more attention is to be given to other resources viz.: soil, irrigation water, nutrients, crops and their management practices to sustain the productivity.

CHAPTER 9

Carbon sequestration in soil

SONALI MAZUMDAR, BIDISHA BANERJEE, R. SINGH *and*
H. PATHAK

*"There is light enough for those who wish to see, and darkness
for those of the opposite disposition."*—Blaise Pascal

CARBON DIOXIDE (CO_2), the principal greenhouse gas, currently accounts for about 60% of the net radiative forcing and has a strong potential to affect current and future climate. Over the past 150 years the amount of carbon in the atmosphere has increased by 30%. In 1992, nearly all countries of the world signed the Framework Convention on Climate Change Agreement, which aimed at stabilizing the atmospheric concentrations of the greenhouse gases especially CO_2. As a step towards this goal, in 1997 international negotiators adopted the Kyoto Protocol to reduce greenhouse gas emissions at the 1990 levels. This emission reduction can be achieved by source and sink improvement. One proposed method to reduce atmospheric CO_2 is to increase the global storage of carbon i.e. by taking CO_2 from the atmosphere via photosynthesis and sequestering it in different components of terrestrial, oceanic, and fresh water aquatic ecosystems. This chapter deals with i) the strategies to sequester carbon in soil and ii) the constraints encountered in soil carbon sequestration.

CARBON SEQUESTRATION

Carbon is found in all living organisms and is the major building block for life on earth. It exists in many forms, predominantly as plant biomass, soil organic matter and as the gas CO_2 in the atmosphere and dissolved in seawater. Under the Framework Convention on Climate Change, a source is any *"process or activity which releases a greenhouse gas, or aerosol or a precursor of a greenhouse gas into the atmosphere"*. A sink is any process, activity or mechanism which removes these from the atmosphere.

Carbon sequestration is, therefore, defined as the capture and secure storage of carbon that would otherwise be emitted to or remains in the atmosphere (FAO, 2000). It generally implies the long-term storage of carbon in the terrestrial biosphere, underground, or the oceans so that the build up of carbon dioxide concentration in the atmosphere will reduce or slow.

Terrestrial biosphere can help in sequestering C through CO_2 removal from the atmosphere by vegetation and storage in biomass and soils. Plants assimilate carbon through photosynthesis and return some of it to the atmosphere through respiration. The carbon that remains as plant tissue is then consumed by animals or added to the soil as litter when plants die and decompose. The primary form that carbon is stored in the soil is as soil organic matter (SOM), which is a complex mixture of carbon compounds, consisting of decomposing plant and animal tissue, microbes (protozoa, nematodes, fungi, and bacteria), and carbon associated with soil minerals. Soil organic matter which plays a vital role in improving soil physical (water holding capacity, porosity etc.), chemical and biological properties is so valuable, it can be referred to as "black gold". Increasing soil C storage can increase infiltration and fertility, decrease wind and water erosion, minimize compaction, enhance water quality, decrease C emissions, impede pesticide movement and enhance environmental quality.

OPTIONS OF CARBON SEQUESTRATION IN AGRICULTURAL SOILS

Soil management practices like increasing soil organic carbon content, reduced tillage, manuring, residue incorporation, improving soil biodiversity, micro aggregation, and mulching can play important roles in sequestering carbon in soil (Figure 1). Strategies to sequester carbon in soils also include increase of (i) total soil organic carbon content, (ii) sub-soil organic carbon content, (iii) microaggregation and (iv) biodiversity. Improved management techniques have shown that scientific agriculture can be a solution to these environmental issues in general and specifically to mitigating the greenhouse effect by increasing soil carbon storage and effectively removing CO_2 from the atmosphere (Figure 2 and 3). Many long-term experiments have demonstrated that judicious applications of fertilizer with appropriate crop rotations and conservation tillage produce the optimum biomass yield and lead to C sequestration in agricultural soils.

Soil organic carbon in the sub soil can be increased by growing crops with deep root systems for transferring carbon to the sub soil and deep ploughing for incorporation of residue in the sub-soil. Increasing the proportion of soil microaggregates by using long-chain polymers, soil condi-

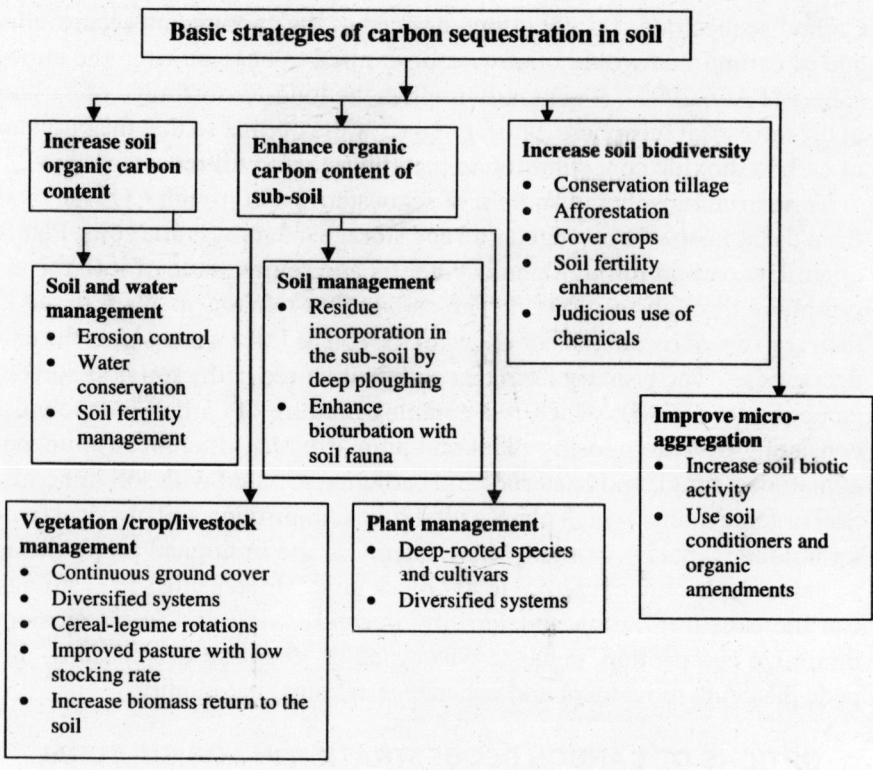

Figure 1: Strategies for carbon sequestration in soils (Lal *et al.*, 1995)

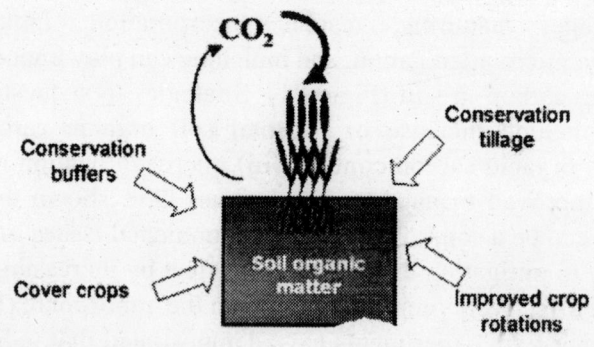

Figure 2: Effects of agricu̶   ̶on balance (Paustian, 2002)

tioners and earthworms
immobilized in such or
ganisms. Besides this
composition of fresh
from agricultural soi

quantities of carbon. Carbon
xes is inaccessible to microor-
tion helps in limiting the de-
educes carbon dioxide emission
ration of atmospheric carbon di-

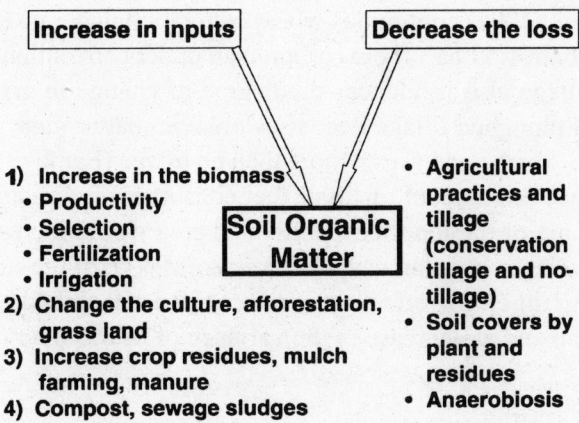

Figure 3: Management of soil organic matter in agriculture

oxide in the soil, ultimately as stable humus, may prove a lasting solution than sequestring carbon dioxide in the standing biomass through reforestration and afforestation (Batjes, 1998).

Besides sequestring carbon by manipulation of soil porperties and by adopting suitable cultivation practices, it can also be increased by keeping less fertile land uncultivated. Uncultivated saline-sodic soils which have carbon mass of 17.7 Gt, lose 4.6 Gt C on cultivation (Mosier, 1998). Therefore, leaving such land as fallow will help in sequestring C and will also save the cost of soil reclamation. Such a suggestion is sound, provided we impress upon increasing the productivity of more fertile land to compensate for the loss of crop yield from less fertile land when left fallow for carbon sequestration. Now, we shall discuss these management practices individually.

Conservation tillage

Intensive tillage especially ploughing accentuates mineralizaton and CO_2 emissions by mixing crop residues into the soil, bringing it closer to microbes, increasing the O_2 concentrations in the soil, and disrupting aggregates and exposing physically protected organic matter to microbial and enzyme activity. Therefore, reducing the intensity and frequency of ploughing and adoption of conservation tillage practices are important strategies for enhancing soil organic carbon (SOC) content. Conservation tillage is a tillage designed to maintain roughness of a field surface and leave most of the previous crop residues on the surface while providing a suitable seed-bed and weed control for the next crop. The roughness reduces run-off, water and wind erosion, thereby improving water use efficiency and increasing carbon concentrations in the topsoil. According to

Campbell *et al.* (1995) continuous wheat cultivation under no tillage condition gained about 1.5 t ha^{-1} more carbon than under conventional condition. Method of tillage also influences the degree of change in organic matter. Mould board ploughed tillage decreases organic matter more than stubble mulch tillage, which decreases it more than no tillage (Lamb *et al.*, 1985). It can also reduce the amount of fossil fuel consumption during farm operations. No tillage of the long-term cultivated area would increase the mean and reduce variance of mean weight diameter (MWD) of the cultivated soil. Conversely no till crop production of never-tilled soil should result in a decrease in mean and an increase in the variance of MWD over time.

Cover crops

The effectiveness of conservation tillage in soil organic carbon sequestration is enhanced by the use of cover crops, such as clover and small grains for protection and soil improvement between periods of regular crop production. These crops improve carbon sequestration by enhancing soil structure, and adding organic matter to the soil. Frequent use of sod-type legumes and grasses in rotation with food crops is an important strategy to enhance SOC and improve soil quality.

Crop rotation

Crop rotation is a sequence of crops grown in regularly recurring succession on the same area of land. It mimics the diversity of natural ecosystems more closely than intensive mono-cropping practices. Varying the type of crops grown can increase the level of soil organic matter. However, effectiveness of crop rotation depends on the type of crops and crop rotation times. Chander *et al.* (1997) studied soil organic matter under different crop rotations for 6 years and found that inclusion of green manure crop of *Sesbania aculeta* improved soil organic matter status. Microbial biomass C increased from 192 mg kg^{-1} soil in pearl millet-wheat fallow rotation to 256 mg kg^{-1} soil in pearl millet wheat green manure rotation. Green manuring improves the soil organic carbon status which in turn improves the soil microbial activity vital for nutrient turnover and long term productivity of the soil. Plant species affect SOC through differences in the amount and depth distribution of root biomass, root respiration, timing and level of root exudates, lignin content, coarse particulate organic matter, soil aggregation and soil biodiversity.

Incorporation of crop residue in soil

Recycling of crop residues, instead of burning, is very crucial for C sequestration as it improves soil organic C content, biological activity, soil structure, infiltration, soil water storage, decreases bulk density and the potential for wind and water erosion (Aulakh and Doran, 2002). The increased soil organic matter leads to increased crop production. Therefore, more CO_2 will be used by the crops and more carbon will be stored in the soil. The increase in SOC content through crop residue application depends on the quantity and quality of the residue, soil properties and management.

Soil fertility and nutrient management

Application of crop residues and other biomass with a wide C:N *per se* is not enough for C sequestration. There is also a need for application of nutrients especially N, P and S. Soil fertility and nutrient management, therefore, has two objectives: (a) supply nutrients for plant growth and development, and (b) supply nutrients for conversion of biomass with high C:N (as much as 100:1) to humus with a low C:N (10:1). On a long-term basis, increased crop yield and organic matter returned to the soil with judicious fertilizer application result in higher SOC content and biological activity than under controlled conditions (absence of fertilizers). A study conducted by Ryan *et al.* (1998) showed that amount of organic matter increased with increasing rates of N fertilizers (0-90 kg ha^{-1}). Application of P fertilizers and phosphoric acids favours aggregation, which buffers soil carbon in micro-aggregates and protects against decomposition. Addition of organic amendments like manure also promotes soil carbon sequestration by adding carbon directly. Besides this application of sewage and sludge enable crop growth and lead to improvements in SOC content.

Liming

Improving soil structure by enhancing aggregation leads to increased SOC content. Liming acid soils can enhance aggregation as Ca^{2+} has strong binding effect on clay particles. When applied in sufficient quantity, Ca^{2+} acts as a binding agent leading to improvement in soil structure.

Water management

In addition to supplemental irrigation, *in situ* soil-water management, particularly in arid and semi-arid regions where crop growth is severely limited by water deficit even if nutrient availability is adequate, is important to enhancing productivity and SOC content of soil. Water harvesting techniques and micro catchments are extremely beneficial in increasing biomass production in arid climates. It has been estimated that the conversion of dryland farming to irrigated agriculture may increase SOC content in the soil profile by 50 to 150 kg ha^{-1} yr^{-1} (Lal *et al.,* 1999).

Elimination of summer fallows

Summer fallowing is often practised in semi arid regions. This practice reduces SOC content of soil by decreasing inputs of plant residues, increasing decomposition rates, and increasing soil erosion. Eliminating summer fallow, therefore, improves carbon sequestration in dryland cropping systems.

LAND CONVERSION AND RESTORATION

The basic strategy in land conversion and restoration is to convert marginal agricultural land to non-agricultural restorative uses (e.g. grassland, forest or wetland).

Cropland to grassland

Placing cultivated or highly erodible land into permanent plant cover like grassland potentially increases the amount of atmospheric CO_2 captured and sequestered as SOC. Establishment of a permanent grass cover can increase the mass of C added into the soil, relative to what may be returned by traditional cropping systems, while lack of mechanical disturbance and absence of tillage decreases rates of SOC oxidation to CO_2 and the rate at which CO_2-C is returned to the atmosphere.

Conservation buffer

Conservation buffers are vegetative filter strips ranging from 5 to 50 m wide, usually are installed along streams to minimize soil erosion, has a good potential for C accumulation.

Restoring wetland

Natural wetlands have a potential to accumulate peat at the rate of 25 to 43 g C m^{-2}yr^{-1} (Mitsch and Wu, 1995). Conversion of natural wetlands to croplands and other urban uses results in reduced carbon storage, therefore, restoring them would promote C sequestration.

Recovery of degraded lands

Soil degradation may be due to several processes, including accelerated soil erosion, salinization, drastic disturbances by mining and urban activities, overstocking and grazing land, decline in soil structure by vehicular traffic and soil contamination by industrial pollutants. Problem of soil degradation is more severe in tropics than in temperate regions. Restoration of these soils is a high priority for economic and environmental reasons. Environmentally, restoration of biological productivity of soils will improve water quality by reducing transport of sediments and sediment borne pollutants, and mitigate greenhouse effect by C immobilization in the biomass and sequestering in soil. Soil erosion management, afforestation and conversion to improved pastures are important strategies. The rate of carbon sequestration through soil restoration depends on antecedent properties, restorative measures, ecoregional characteristics, and the initial SOC pool under natural conditions.

Afforestation

Afforestation of marginal and degraded lands can help in reducing loss of soil and at the same time improve SOC status. The Intergovernmental Panel on Climate Change's (IPCC) second assessment report found that during the period 1995–2050, slowing deforestation, promoting natural forest regeneration, and encouraging global reforestation could offset 220–320 billion tons of CO_2 (12–15%) of fossil emissions. Forests store carbon in woody tissues and soil organic matter. The net rate of carbon uptake is greatest when forests are young, and slows with time. When forests are cut, the carbon they contain may be quickly returned to the atmosphere if the woody tissue is burned or converted to products, such as paper, that are short-lived. If the wood is used for construction or furniture, then those products retain carbon during their life-times and act as carbon sinks. They have positive secondary environmental benefits, such as restoration of degraded lands and protection of biodiversity, as well as social benefits, such as employing indigenous people through tree planting programmes.

Restoration of pastures and rangeland

Rangelands make up the most extensive terrestrial ecosystem on the planet. Perennial grasses, a major component of most rangeland plant communities, enhance C storage into the soil as grasses have a much higher portion of total plant biomass in below ground tissues than do trees, most shrubs, or annual crops. Most rangeland ecosystems evolved under grazing by large herbivores, and for these ecosystems, grazing appears to be a necessary component to overall health of the ecosystem. Developing livestock grazing strategies that optimize the stability and diversity of the plant community will optimize soil C sequestration.

ESTIMATION OF C SEQUESTRATION POTENTIAL IN SOIL

Direct measurement of C sequestration over time is to measure sequential changes in soil carbon. Such measurements are complicated by the spatial and temporal heterogenity of soil carbon contents. This problem can be overcome through the use of well-designed sampling and analysis procedures and use of simulation modelling. Mathematical modelling of soil carbon sequestration is relatively well developed particularly for agricultural soils. Models are used to determine the variation and changes in SOC content across different regions and with various management practices. Some models simulate crop growth and residue inputs directly, while others require that organic matter addition rates be specified as model inputs. The important models in C dynamics are CENTURY, DNDC, DAISY, OBM, NCSWAP, BOX, etc. The use of soil organic matter models range from the field level to regional and global applications. The data obtained is adjusted for local conditions using Geographical Information Systems (GIS) databases. Use of simulation models in conjunction with field level experiments and GIS for its verification are promising.

CONSTRAINTS TO CARBON SEQUESTRATION IN SOIL

Achieving net greenhouse gas emission offsets requires change in agricultural operations. Many of the strategies divert land or inputs away from crop or possibly timber production. On the agricultural side crop prices generally rise while production falls. Exports also are strongly affected. Sustainable forest management may lead to increased rotation age and decreased timber harvesting which affect global timber market forcing timber companies in developing countries to undertake deforestation. Conversion of cropland to grassland reduces food yield. It must be compensated somewhere else to feed exploding population. So the farmers will be forced to adopt drastic measures to augment yield from their farmlands. The need to reduce emissions and implementations of emissions trading will also affect fossil fuel prices. The tax and corresponding transportation costs increase and might influence the cost of petrol based agriculture chemicals and fertilizers as well as price of on and off-farm commodities. Carbon sequestration in the agricultural soils is permanent as long as the farmers use the procedures of conservation agriculture. However, the transition to conservation agriculture is neither spontaneous nor free of cost. There may be extra costs for some tools or equipment. Besides this shifting to conservation tillage from conventional will result in reduced rate of mineralization, high fertilizer and herbicide requirement and more pollution problems. Leaving crop residues on soil surface will delay the sowing of next crop since a certain time is required for their decomposition. Apart from this it causes pest and disease infestation. Some practices such as increasing soil fertility via nitrogen fertilization could lead to increased primary productivity and increased carbon storage, but it could also lead to increase in nitrous oxide emission. Also, by increasing soil water content the rates of decomposition will decrease but methane production could increase. As the soil carbon level increases, soil absorption of carbon decreases and soil potential to become a future emission source increases. Subsequent alteration of the management regime can lead to carbon releases. Therefore, adoption of any management practice should be carried out after prior evaluation of its overall effect.

Despite all the beneficial effects of carbon sequestration on agriculture and environment there are several constraints in its implementation. Various management practices discussed in this chapter increase SOC content but they are still not popular among the farmers. Successful and lasting change needs land users working in association and some initial investment. In this connection, new strategies and appropriate policies must be developed. Policy intervention in both the public and private sectors is necessary to realize a significant amount of this carbon sequestration potential. Policy tools with the potential to promote increased soil carbon sequestration include carbon credit trading, incentives for development and application of new technologies, education and technical assistance for producers, and tax credits for conservation practices. Based on this set of criteria, carbon credit trading stands in the forefront as the most promising policy option. The Kyoto Protocol provides the mechanisms that would allow transfers or crediting of emissions reductions achieved in other countries through joint implementation (JI), clean development mechanism (CDM) and credits or allowances through international emissions trading.

Through proper management, organic matter content of most soils with low organic carbon can be increased, therefore, the potential to sequester carbon in soil around the world through soil management is significant. But managing soil at the global scale is by no means simple or even practical, because many social, economical, political and technological barriers exist. By understanding the processes and factors that affect sequestration of carbon in soil, soil management is more effectively utilized to maintain soil carbon stock or increase carbon sequestration in soil. However, it is unlikely that soil alone can provide a large enough sink for carbon to offset total increase in atmospheric carbon dioxide and other greenhouse gases. A coordinated effort both at the national and international levels is needed to facilitate adoption of technologies that enhance food production, increase soil carbon pool and improve environment.

CHAPTER 10

Mitigation of nitrous oxide emission from soil

H. Pathak, V. Sharma, Arti Bhatia *and* P. K. Singh

"A sustainable society is one, which satisfies its needs without diminishing the prospects of future generations."
—Lester R. Brown

S OIL CONTRIBUTES SIGNIFICANTLY TOWARDS nitrous oxide emission to the atmosphere. It is a by-product of nitrification and an intermediate product of denitrification process (Chapter 3). There are no significant sinks or uptake mechanisms of nitrous oxide in soil systems. Therefore, the mitigation should focus entirely on emission reduction. There are two major strategies to mitigate nitrous oxide emission from soil: a) to influence land-use management practices in case of intensive agricultural systems and b) to influence the land-use in extensive agricultural systems.

MITIGATION OF NITROUS OXIDE EMISSION IN INTENSIVE AGRICULTURAL SYSTEMS

Intensive agricultural systems, envisaging high productivity, high input use, high rainfall or irrigated systems, are widely recognized as major sources of nitrous oxide emission. It is argued that there is substantial scope of mitigating nitrous oxide emission from such systems. Appropriate crop management practices, which lead to increased N-use efficiency and higher yield by optimizing the crop's natural ability to compete with the N-loss processes hold the key to mitigate nitrous oxide emission. The various approaches to increase N-use efficiency (Figure 1) and their nitrous oxide emission mitigation potential (Table 1) have been discussed below.

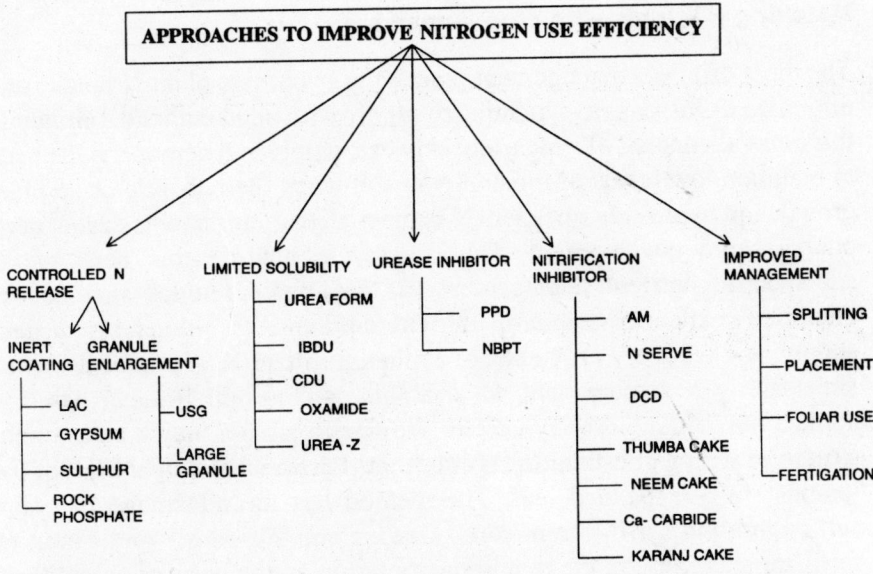

Figure 1: Approaches to improve nitrogen use efficiency and reducing nitrous oxide emission (*Source*: Pathak *et al.*, 1998)

Table 1. Strategies to mitigate nitrous oxide emission from agricultural soils

Management practices	Decrease in emission (Tg N yr⁻¹)
1. Matching N supply with crop demand	0.24
a. Use soil/plant testing to determine fertilizers need	
b. Minimize fallow periods to limit mineral N accumulation	
c. Optimize split application schemes	
d. Match N application to reduce production goals in regions of crop over production	
2. Tightening N flow cycles	0.14
a. Integrate animal and crop production systems in terms of manure reuse in crop production	
b. Maintaining plant residue N on the production site	
3. Use of advanced fertilization techniques	0.15
a. Controlled release of fertilizers	
b. Place fertilizers below the soil surface	
c. Foliar application of fertilizers	
d. Use nitrification inhibitors	
e. Match fertilizer type to seasonal precipitation	
4. Optimizing tillage, irrigation and drainage	0.15
Total	0.68

Source: Mosier *et al.* (1998)

Matching N supply with crop demand

The most efficient management practice to maximize plant N uptake and minimize its losses is to synchronize supply with plant demand. Implicit in this general concept of synchrony between supply and demand is the need to maintain low levels of mineral N in soil when there is little or no plant growth and to provide sufficient N to meet plant requirements during periods of rapid development. The strategy to achieve this objective is site-specific nutrient management (SSNM) that includes site-specific quantitative knowledge of crop nutrient requirements, indigenous nutrient supply, and recovery efficiency of applied fertilizer N. A practical way of site-specific N management, for example, is chlorophyll meter-based N application. The chlorophyll meter provides a simple, quick and nondestructive method of estimating N concentration on a dry weight basis of the topmost fully expanded leaf. The method has the advantage of being self-calibrating for different soils, seasons and varieties. Application of fertilizer according to the requirement of crop on the basis of chlorophyll meter reading increases the fertilizer use efficiency because of less fertilizer application. As a consequence less accumulation of mineral forms of N (NH_4^+ and NO_3^-) within the crop root zone and hence less losses of N and nitrous oxide emission. Recently a simple tool, leaf colour chart, has been introduced to measure the greenness of the leaves and guide the requirement of N application (Figure 2). The practice is being promoted with the farmers and holds a good promise in increasing N-use efficiency.

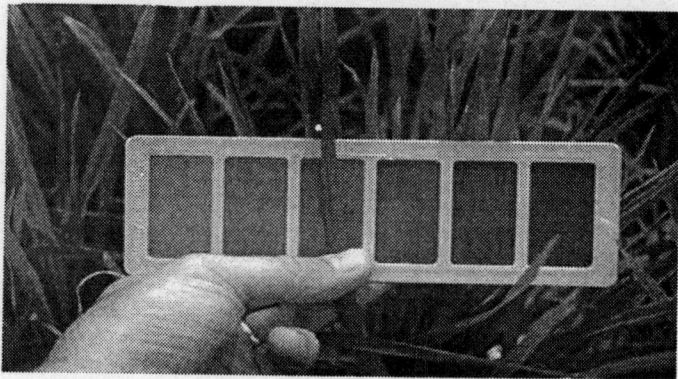

Figure 2: Matching N supply with crop demand using leaf colour chart

Using proper fertilizer formulation

The form of added N plays an important role in regulating nitrous oxide emission. The amount of nitrous oxide evolved from soil treated with ammonium sulphate [$(NH_4)_2SO_4$] or urea (NH_2CONH_2) is significantly more than from those soil which receive the same amount of nitrogen as calcium nitrate [$Ca(NO_3)_2$]. It has also been observed that the nitrous oxide emission is larger from soils fertilized with anhydrous ammonia than from those fertilized with nitrate and ammonium salts (Duxbury *et al.*, 1982). Studies at the Indian Agricultural Research Institute have shown that urea, which is widely used as a nitrogenous fertilizer in the country, contributes maximum to the nitrous oxide emission. It is followed by ammonium sulphate, ammonium chloride and potassium nitrate from alluvial soil at field capacity moisture regimes (Majumdar *et al.*, 2000). Applications of nitrate (NO_3-N) fertilizers, such as calcium ammonium nitrate (CAN), in crops with aerobic conditions and of ammonium (NH_4-N) fertilizers, such as ammonium sulphate, urea, etc. in wetland crops, therefore, help in reducing the emission.

By using controlled release fertilizer to release N in synchrony with plant growth it should be possible to provide sufficient N in a single application to satisfy plant requirements. With this concept, gaseous loss would be small because of the limited substrate. Many different slow-release forms of N have been suggested for application but their adoption by the farmers was poor because of extra cost involved and less marginal profit.

Method of application

Nitrous oxide emission not only depends on the type of fertilizer nitrogen used but also on the mode of its application. The application of urea in plough layers gives less emission of nitrous oxide than broadcast application of urea fertilizer. The emission of different amounts of nitrous oxide from different forms of fertilizer nitrogen suggests that controlling this factor is an efficient way of limiting the emission. Addition of phosphorus and liming materials can also affect nitrous oxide evolution from soil. However, phosphorus induced emissions are higher than those obtained with lime. Plant uptake of fertilizer N can be improved by various methods of application such as deep placement and placing fertilizer in bands, thereby minimizing the loss of N and mitigating nitrous oxide emission.

It is generally agreed that more efficient use of fertilizer N results when application of fertilizer coincides with the period of rapid plant uptake. Several application of small amounts of fertilizer N during the growing season have proven more useful for supplying N for plant growth in some systems than one large dose at the beginning of the season. Unfortunately, multiple applications of fertilizer are not always practical in many agricultural situations because of the precipitation patterns, extra cost and difficulty in applying fertilizer within a maturing crop canopy.

When irrigation is used, there is opportunity for supplying fertilizer N along with the irrigation water. This allows the farmer to overcome some of the limitations in supplying multiple applications of fertilizer N to crops by conventional techniques and to tune fertilizer N supply to crop requirements. Nitrogen can be supplied by dissolving fertilizer in the water applied to crops in sprinkler systems, or by furrow and flood irrigation. This method has the advantages of simplicity, convenience and low cost and has been found to increase N-use efficiency.

Foliar fertilization is one way of supplying N during periods of rapid plant growth and N demand, or at times of critical physiological stress. It has been used successfully for late applications of N to cereal, leguminous and fibre crops to increase grain protein and yield. Direct measurement of gaseous emission in such systems showed that very little N was lost from foliar applied urea unless rainfall washed unassimilated urea from the plant onto the soil.

Use of N-transformation inhibitors

Nitrogen use efficiency could be increased by retarding the hydrolysis of urea to ammonia by the use of urease inhibitors or by regulating nitrate accumulation by nitrification inhibitors. This results in the reduction of direct nitrous oxide emission from nitrifiers, and reduces the availability of NO_3^-, necessary for denitrification (Prasad and Power, 1995). Nitrapyrin, acetylene, dicyandiamide (DCD), 2-amino-4-chloro–6-methyl-pyrimidine (AM) and 2-sulphanilamide-thiazole (ST) are some of the promising nitrification inhibitors in agriculture and have also been found effective in reducing nitrous oxide emission from soils (Pathak and Nedwell, 2001). Similarly, wax-coated calcium carbide and ATC (4-amino 1,2,4-triazole) reduce the rate of nitrification and hence, the emission of nitrous oxide. Most of these nitrification inhibitors, however, have limitations. For example, the efficacy of the most commonly used nitrification inhibitor nitrapyrin gets reduced due to sorption on soil colloids, hydrolysis and loss through volatilization. It has been established in laboratory studies that acetylene is a potent inhibitor of nitrification (Bremner and Blackmer, 1979), but because being in the gaseous state at ambient temperature there are problems in introducing it during the growing period at the concentration required to limit nitrification. This problem may be overcome by the use of calcium carbide coated with layers of wax and shellac to provide a slow-release source of acetylene (Banerjee and Mosier, 1989). Another way of overcoming the problem of applying gaseous acetylene is to use substituted acetylenes such as 2-ethynylpyridine or phenylacetylene, which are liquids at ambient temperatures. Another nitrification inhibitor,

DMPP (3,4-Dimethyl pyrazole phosphate) decreases the release of nitrous oxide by 49%. Pathak and Nedwell (2001) found that in the presence of Nitrapyrin, AM, and DCD emission of nitrous oxide was reduced by 12, 24 and 63%, respectively, where as sodium thiosulphate, sulphur, thiourea and acetylene had no effect on emission of nitrous oxide. Under submerged conditions, no inhibitor remains effective in reducing nitrous oxide emission. There are some plant-derived organics such as neem oil and neem cake, which can act as nitrification inhibitors. These are being experimented in the fields to find their efficacy in reducing the emission of nitrous oxide and increasing the fertilizer-use efficiency. Some biocidal inhibitors, such as karanja seed extract, have been found to retard nitrification by 60-70% (Majumdar *et al.*, 2001). The effect of various nitrification inhibitors along with urea application has been shown in Table 2.

Table 2. Reduction of nitrous oxide emission with nitrification inhibitors

Treatment	*Wheat*	*Corn*	*Ryegrass*	*Rice*
	N_2O-N emission (g ha^{-1})			
Urea	930	1650	2700	59.9
Urea + DCD	440	—	1000	49.0
Urea + coated Ca-carbide	510	480	—	—
Urea + Nitrapyin	—	980	1500	—
Unfertilized soil	440	110	—	34.3

Source: Mosier *et al.* (1996)

However, for inhibitors to be successful following criteria should be fulfilled (Mosier *et al.*, 1998): (a) urease activity or nitrification must be inhibited until the fertilizer penetrates the soil surface or mineral N derived from it is assimilated by plants, (b) gaseous emissions in the field must be reduced, (c) crop or forage yield must be increased, (d) inhibitors must cost less than the N lost by NH_3 volatilization or denitrification, and (e) inhibitors must be capable of being incorporated with the fertilizer N, be stable during manufacture and storage and be environmentally safe. The general lack of availability and cost effectiveness of such inhibitors in the developing world prohibits their use.

Optimize irrigation and drainage

Irrigation should be provided as and when required so as to increase the N use efficiency and reduce the emission of nitrous oxide. Moreover, applying water as needed saves both water and energy for pumping. Various technologies like drip irrigation, sprinkler irrigation, use of soil moisture sensors to predict irrigation requirement have immense potential in increasing water and N-use efficiencies.

Crop cultivars

Crop cultivars with a) low emission, b) high N-use efficiency, c) faster decomposition of residues and d) less water-demanding have potential to reduce nitrous oxide emission from soil.

Optimize tillage operation

Optimizing tillage practices including a) no-tillage or minimum tillage, b) bed planting, c) reducing compaction and d) improving drainage also help in mitigating the nitrous oxide emission from soil by less soil disturbance, and high N and water-use efficiencies.

MITIGATION OF NITROUS OXIDE EMISSION IN EXTENSIVE AGRICULTURAL SYSTEMS

Extensive agriculture systems are characterized by low productivity, low input use operated in poor soil and low rainfall areas and are used for grazing and shifting cultivation. In response to declining agricultural yields and population pressures, farmers in many regions regularly convert forests to cropping land, and many of their techniques involve burning. Shifting cultivation requires that forests be cut, logging debris and unwanted vegetation burned, and the land farmed for several years and then left fallow to revegenate. Savanna and rangeland biomass is often burned to improve livestock forage. Following methods could be promoted in order to make extensive agriculture more viable and sustainable and in mitigating the nitrous oxide emission (Mosier *et al.,* 1998).

- Land use change
  — Conversion of marginal crop land area to grassland or trees
  — Replacing annual or seasonal crops with tree crops, where possible
  — Minimize fallow periods by growing cover crops

- Increasing the productivity of agricultural land
  — Optimizing crop management
  — Optimize irrigation and drainage
  — Optimize fertilizer use
  — Reclamation of problem soils

- Lengthening the rotation times and improving the productivity of shifted agriculture

- Increasing grassland management
- Recycling of crop residues into soil
- Increasing use of crop residues as household fuel
- Maintain soil pH above 5
- Use of N-fixing crops
- Prevent soil compaction

IMPLEMENTATION OF MITIGATION STRATEGIES

The implementation of mitigation strategies requires decisions at many different levels.

- *International (International Organizations):* Various UN organizations and NGO's will have to work with the local bodies and the Government of concerned states in a compatible manner to implement the mitigation strategies.
- *National (National Governments):* At National Government levels, following steps should be taken: a) land use should be determined by *Climate Policy* along with *Agriculture Policy*, b) taking away some land area from agricultural production e.g. Government set-aside programs, c) public education programs to help advance adoption, d) crop insurance to share the risk of failure, e) providing subsidy to popularize nitrification inhibitors and f) fixing quotas to limit N use.
- *Local (Local bodies):* The implementation work has to be started from the root level with the help of local institutions. The participation from these bodies is must in order to implementing these strategies successfully.
- *Field (Farmer's) level:* At farmer's level initiatives can be carried out for a) rationalization of fertilizer use, b) switching of cultivars, c) use of slow release fertilizers and inhibitors, d) residue recycling and e) altering soil conditions.

Potential policy instruments to implement the mitigation options could be as follows:

- Market based options
  — Fertilizer tax
  — Intervention (area payments, set aside, quotas)
  — Removing subsidy
  — Incentives to agri-environment management

- Regulation/restrictions
  — Limits of N application

  — Nitrate vulnerable zones
  — Restrictions of straw burning

- Enhancing the knowledge-base
  — Technology transfer
  — Awareness
  — Funding of scientific research

Agriculture, including forestry, has been proposed as a relatively cheap source of net emission reductions. The economic impacts on agriculture of these policies to reduce greenhouse gas emissions depend on the intensity of mitigation efforts, the efficiency of emission markets, and the speed of technological developments both in the agricultural and non-agricultural sectors. There is a need to strengthen the mitigation option research for:

- Improving soil and crop management
- Developing new fertilizer and nitrification inhibitors, which are cheap and locally available
- Comprehensive model-based analyses and improved global databases on soils, land use and trace gas fluxes
- Developing varieties with low emission. Genetically engineered plants may have good potential
- Cost/benefit analysis involving local conditions
- Improving assessment of mitigation options
- Developing analytical tools that incorporate socio-economic factors

In conclusion mitigation practices that recover investment cost and generate a profit in the short-term are preferred over practices that require a long-term to recover investment costs. Practices that have a high probability associated with expected profits are desired over practices that have less certainty about their returns. When human resource constraints or knowledge of the practice prevent adoption, public education programs can improve the knowledge and skills of the work force and managers to help advance adoption. Greenhouse gas emission is a complex problem but needs a simple solution, as it has to be adopted by millions of farmers farming in the different parts of the world with different levels of resource availability and agro-climatic conditions. No single approach is suitable for all situations. Therefore, a basket of mitigation options is required. Moreover, there are trade-offs of greenhouse gas emission. Hence attempts should be made for reducing the total quantity rather than individual gas emission. Most importantly the mitigation practice should not have any negative impact on food production, which is the most pressing need in many parts of the world.

CHAPTER 11

International initiatives on combating global warming

JYOTHI KUMARI, AJIT GOVIND *and* H. PATHAK

"How far must suffering and misery go before we see that even in the day of vast cities and powerful machines, the good earth is our mother and that if we destroy her, we destroy ourselves?"—Paul Bigelow Sears

'GLOBAL WARMING' HAS BEEN perceived as a serious threat to the existence of mankind by the International communities. Several steps are being taken worldover to limit the threat of rapid change in global atmosphere and its associated consequences. In 1972, the United Nations Conference on the Human Environment (UNCHE) was held in Stockholm, Sweden. This was the first global conference to focus on negative human impacts on the environment, which led to the formation of United Nations Environment Programe (UNEP). Since then, a number of meetings have been held and these negotiations led to the formation of a number of international organizations and programmes, which have emerged as fora for consideration of environmental problems. A brief description of some of the important organizations is given below:

1. Inter-governmental Panel on Climate Change (IPCC), headquartered in Washington, D.C., was established by the UNEP and WMO in November 1988 to assess the scientific, technical and socio-economic information relevant to the understanding of the risk of human induced climate change. It does not carry out research nor does it monitor climate related data or other relevant parameters. IPCC bases its assessment mainly on peer-reviewed and published scientific/technical literature. IPCC has three working groups and a taskforce: (i) Working Group I assesses the scientific aspects of the climate system and climate change, (ii) Working Group II addresses the vulnerability of socio-economic and natural systems to climate change, and (iii) Working Group III assesses options for limiting greenhouse gas emissions and otherwise mitigating climate change. The Taskforce on National Greenhouse Gas inventories is responsible for the IPCC National Greenhouse Gas Inventories Programme. So far IPCC has published three assessment reports (1990, 1995, 2001).

2. United Nations Environment Programme (UNEP), established in 1972, works to encourage sustainable development through sound environmental practices. Its activities cover a wide range of issues, from atmosphere and terrestrial ecosystems, the promotion of environmental science and information, to an early warning and emergency response capacity to deal with environmental disasters and emergencies. UNEP is headquartered in Nairobi, Kenya, and has regional and outposted offices in Paris, Geneva, Osaka, The Hague, Washington, New York, Bangkok, Mexico City, Manama, Montreal and Bonn. The mission statement of the UNEP is "to provide leadership and encourage partnership in caring for the environment by inspiring, informing and enabling nations and peoples to improve their quality of life without compromising that of the future generations".

3. The Intergovernmental Negotiating Committee for a Framework Convention on Climate Change (INC/FCCC): By 1990, numerous international conferences had issued urgent calls for a binding global treaty that addressed the problems of climate change. Then an inter-governmental working group was formed by UNEP and WMO (World meteorological Organization) to prepare for climate treaty negotiations. The UN General Assembly confirmed this proposal in 1990 and set up the INC to draft a framework convention and prepare a legally binding climate treaty. The United Nations Framework Convention on Climate Change (UNFCCC) is the first binding international legal instrument that deals directly with climate change. The Convention was adopted on 9 May 1992. It was opened for signature at the "Earth Summit" in Rio de Janeiro the following month, where it was signed by the representatives of 154 states. By 19 June 1993, when the treaty was closed for signature, 165 states (plus the EEC) had signed the treaty. The 50th ratification was received on 21 December 1993, triggering the Convention's entry into force 90 days later on 21 March 1994. The Convention's ultimate objective is the "stabilization of greenhouse gas concentrations in the atmosphere at a level that would prevent dangerous anthropogenic interference with the climate system". As a framework treaty, the convention sets out principles and general commitments, leaving more specific obligations to future legal instruments. The key principles incorporated in the treaty are the precautionary principles, the common but differentiated responsibility of states, and the importance of sustainable development (Article 3). The general commitments, which apply to both developed and developing countries, are to adopt national programmes for mitigating climate change; to develop adaptation strategies; to promote the sustainable management and conservation of greenhouse gas "sinks" (such as forests); to take climate change into account when setting relevant social, economic, and environmental policies; to co-operate in technical, scientific, and educational matters; and to promote scientific research and the exchange of information .

4. The United Nations Conference on Environment and Development (UNCED) was held in Rio de Janeiro on June 3-14, 1992. This so-called Earth Summit took place 20 years after the 1972 Stockholm Declaration first laid the foundations of contemporary environmental policy. As a high-level forum with universal participation, UNCED's main aim was to show the way to a new global strategy for reconciling development needs with environmental protection. The key results of UNCED were the Rio Declaration, Agenda 21, Forest Principles, and two international conventions concerning climate change and biodiversity.

5. World Meterological Organization (WMO) is involved in activities from weather prediction to air pollution research, climate change related activities, ozone layer depletion studies and tropical storm forecasting. The World Meteorological Organization coordinates global scientific activity to allow increasingly prompt and accurate weather information and other services for public, private and commercial use. WMO's activities contribute to the safety of life and property, the socio-economic development of nations and the protection of the environment. Within the United Nations, the Geneva-based 185-Member Organization provides the authoritative scientific voice on the state and behaviour of the Earth's atmosphere and climate.

7. Advanced International Studies Unit (AISU), based in Washington D.C. is a part of Atmospheric Sciences and Global Change in the Fundamental Science Division of the Pacific Northwest National Laboratory operated by Battelle for the U.S. Department of Energy. AISU has three sets of goals: (i) Global: reducing the threat of climate change and other gobal environmental problems, (ii) National: providing support to economies in transition and emerging democracies, and (iii) Local: Helping local governments meet the needs of their citizens while reducing pollution and saving money.

8. Global Environment Facility (GEF) was established to forge international co-operation and finance actions to address the critical threats to the global environment and to promote environmentally sound and sustainable economic development. It was created in agreement between the

World Bank, UNEP and UNDP comprising 166 member governments, leading development institutions, the scientific communities and non-governmental organizations. *Sources*: (i) www.pnl.gov.\aisu\ (ii) www.wmo-ch\ (iii) www.unep.org\ (iv) www.unfec.int\

Several other organizations are working on climate change. Some of the prominent organizations and programmes are listed below:

AGO	Australian Greenhouse Office
AMAP	Arctic Monitoring and Assessment Programme
ANZECC	Australian and New Zealand Environment and Conservation Council
ANZMEC	Australian and New Zealand Minerals and Energy Council
APN	Asia-Pacific Network for Global Change Research
AusAID	Australian Agency for International Development
CASE	International Centre for Application of Solar Energy
CASID	The Center for Advanced Study of International Development
CCME	Canadian Council of Ministers of the Environment
CCPA	Canadian Centre for Policy Alternatives
CDIAC	Carbon Dioxide Information Analysis Center
CEDAR	Central European Environmental Data Request Facility
CELA	Canadian Environmental Law Association
CESD	Commissioner of the Environment and Sustainable Development
CETAC	Canadian Environmental Technology Advancement Corporation
CGCP	Canadian Global Change Program
CGER	Center for Global Environmental Research
CGIAR	Consultative Group on International Agricultural Research
CHS	(UN) Commission on Human Settlements
CIDA	Canadian International Development Agency
CIER	Centre for Indigenous Environmental Resources
CIESIN	Consortium for International Earth Science Information Network
CIF	Canadian Institute of Forestry
CITES	(UN) Convention on the International Trade of Endangered Species
COAG	Council of Australian Governments
CODATA	Committee on Data for Science and Technology
CPD	(UN) Commission on Population & Development

CPPA	Canadian Pulp and Paper Association (Montreal)
CRC	Cooperative Research Centre
CRRI	Central Rice Research Institute
CSE	Centre for Science and Environment
CSERGE	International Social Science Council
CSIRO	Commonwealth Scientific and Industrial Research Organization
CTE	(WTO) Committee on Trade and Environment
CWF	Canadian Wildlife Federation
DESA	(UN) Department for Economic and Social Affairs
DETR	(UK) Department for the Environment, Transport and the Regions
DFAIT	Canada Department of Foreign Affairs and International Trade
DSD	(UN) Division on Sustainable Development
DST	Department of Science and Technology (India)
EAERE	European Association of Environmental and Resource Economists
ECDG XI	European Commission Directorate General XI (Env. & Nuclear Safety)
ECA	(UN) Economic Commission for Africa
ECE	(UN) Economic Commission for Europe
ENRICH	European Network for Research in Global Change
EPA	United States Environmental Protection Agency
ESAA	Electricity Supply Association of Australia
ESCAP	(UN) Economic & Social Commission for Asia & the Pacific
ESCWA	(UN) Economic & Social Commission for Western Asia
FAO	Food and Agriculture Organization of the United Nations
GCTE	Central European Environmental Data Request Facility
GECHS	Global Environmental Change and Human Security project
GEF	Global Environment Facility
GEWEX	Global Energy and Water Cycle Experiment
GFPP	Global Forestry Policy Project
GIPME	Global Investigation of Pollution in the Marine Environment
GPA	Global Programme of Action for the Protection of the Marine Environment from Land-based Activities
GPCC	Global Precipitation Climatology Centre
GRDC	Global Runoff Data Centre
GTI	Global Toxics Institute

HLG	COAG High Level Group on Greenhouse
IACSD	Inter Agency Committee on Sustainable Development
IAEA	International Atomic Energy Agency
IAHS	International Association of Hydrological Sciences
IAI	Inter-American Institute for Global Change Research
IAMAS	International Association of Meteorology and Atmospheric Sciences
ICES	International Council for the Exploration of the Sea
ICFTU	International Confederation of Free Trade Unions
ICHRDD	International Centre for Human Rights and Democratic Development
ICIMOD	International Centre for Integrated Mountain Development
ICLEI	International Centre for Local Environmental Initiatives
ICRAF	International Centre for Research on Agriculture and Forestry
ICSU	International Council of Scientific Unions
ICTSD	International Centre for Trade and Sustainable Development
IDRC	International Development Research Centre
IFAD	International Fund for Agricultural Development
IFAP	International Federation of Agricultural Producers
IFF	Inter-governmental Forum on Forests
IGBP	International Geosphere-Biosphere Programme
IGO	Inter-Governmental Organization
IGOSS	Integrated Global Ocean Services System
IHDP-IT	The International Human Dimensions Programme on Industrial Transformation
IIASA	International Institute for Applied Systems Analysis
IIED	International Institute for Environment and Development
IISD	International Institute for Sustainable Development
IITM	Indian Institute of Tropical Meteorology
IMO	International Maritime Organization
INFOHYDRO	Hydrological Information Referral Service
INFOTERRA	International Environmental Information System
IODE	International Oceanographic Data and Information Exchange
IPCC	Intergovernmental Panel on Climate Change
IPF	Intergovernmental Panel on Forests
IPGRI	International Plant Genetic Resources Institute
IRPP	Institute for Research on Public Policy
ISEE	International Society for Ecological Economics

ISRIC	International Soil Reference and Information Centre
ISSC	International Social Science Council
ITSU	Tsunami Warning System in the Pacific
ITTO	International Tropical Timber Organization
IUCN	International Council for the Conservation of Nature
IULA	International Union of Local Authorities
IWC	International Whaling Commission
IWSA	International Water Services Association
JGOFS	Joint Global Ocean Flux Study
JODC	Japan Oceanographic Data Center
LEAD	Leadership in Environment and Development Foundation
MAB	Man and the Biosphere Programme
MAFF	(UK) Ministry of Fisheries and Food
MRTEE	Manitoba Round Table on the Environment and the Economy
MSC	Marine Stewardship Council
NASA	National Aeronautics and Space Administration
NatHERS	National House Energy Rating Scheme
NATO	North Atlantic Treaty Organization
NCAS	National Carbon Accounting System
NECA	National Electricity Code Administrator
NGGIC	National Greenhouse Gas Inventory Committee
NGLS	United Nations Non-Governmental Liaison Service
NGRP	National Greenhouse Research Program
NHT	Natural Heritage Trust
NIES	National Institute for Environmental Studies
NPL	National Physical Laboratory
OECD	Organization for Economic Co-operation & Development
OEEC	Organization for European Economic Co-operation
PICES	North Pacific Marine Science Organization
QCPTA	Queensland Cleaner Production Task Force Association
REC	The Regional Environmental Center for the Central and Eastern Europe
REIIF	Renewable Energy Innovation Investment Fund
RMIT	Royal Melbourne Institute of Technology
SEDAC	Socio-economic Data and Applications Center
SEED	Sustainable Energy and socio-economic Data and Applications Center
SEI	Stockholm Environment Institute
SIDS	Small Island Developing States
SPREP	South Pacific Regional Environmental Programme

START	Global Change SysTem for Analysis, Research and Training
TEACOM	Temperate East Asia Regional Committee
TERI	Tata Energy Research Institute
UCCEE	UNEP Collaboration Centre on Energy and Environment
UNCED	United Nations Conference on Environment and Development
UNCHS	United Nations Centre for Human Settlements
UNCLOS	United Nations Convention on the Law of the Seas
UNCSD	United Nations Commission on Sustainable Development
UNCTAD	United Nations Conference on Trade and Development
UNDESA	United Nations Department on Economic & Social Affairs
UNDP	United Nations Development Programme
UNDPCSD	UN Division for Policy Co-ordination for Sustainable Development
UNDSD	United Nations Division for Sustainable Development
UNEP	United Nations Environmental Programme
UNESCO	United Nations Educational, Scientific and Cultural Organization
UNESCO-IOC	UNESCO Inter-governmental Oceanographic Commission
UNFCCC	United Nations Framework Convention on Climate Change
UNICEF	United Nations Children's Emergency Fund
UNIDO	United Nations Industrial Development Organization
UNRISD	United Nations Research Institute for Social Development
USAID	United States Agency for International Development
WBCSD	World Business Council for Sustainable Development
WCDMP	World Climate Data and Monitoring Programme
WCED	World Commission on Environment and Development
WCFSD	World Commission on Forests and Sustainable Development
WCMC	World Conservation Monitoring Centre
WCRP	World Climate Research Programme
WDCGG	The World Data Centre for Greenhouse Gases
WDR	World Development Report
WEC	World Environment Centre
WEO	World Environment Organization
WHO	World Health Organization
WICE	World Industry Council for the Environment

WMO	World Meteorological Organization
WOUDC	World Ozone and Ultraviolet Radiation Data Centre
WREEP	Wholesale/Retail Energy Efficiency Program
WRI	World Resources Institute
WSSD	World Summit for Social Development
WWF	Worldwide Fund for Nature
WWI	World-watch Institute
WWW	World Weather Watch

The implementation of a climate regime depends on the services of these organizations and programmes. The negotiation on climate change only cannot solve the problem but the implementation of the results of these negotiations is necessary. For a successful climate regime, there should be establishment and management of a specialized climate fund. Also, it is necessary to manage the response to concerns about poverty, the issue raised by Late Prime Minister of India Mrs. Indira Gandhi in the United Nations Conference on the Human Environment in Stockholm, Sweden in 1972. Thus, our sustainable future depends upon concerns about poverty, equity, development and climate change.

Glossary

Acid rain   Rainwater that has an acidity content greater than the postulated natural pH of about 5.6. It is formed when sulphur dioxides and nitrogen oxides, as gases or fine particles in the atmosphere, combine with water vapor and precipitate as sulphuric acid or nitric acid in rain, snow, or fog. The dry forms are acidic gases or particulates.

Aerosol   Particulate matter, solid or liquid, larger than a molecule but small enough to remain suspended in the atmosphere. Natural sources include salt particles from sea spray, dust and clay particles as a result of weathering of rocks, both of which are carried upward by the wind. Aerosols can also originate as a result of human activities and are often considered pollutants. Aerosols are important in the atmosphere as nuclei for the condensation of water droplets and ice crystals, as participants in various chemical cycles, and as absorbers and scatterers of solar radiation, thereby influencing the radiation budget of the Earth's climate system.

Air pollution   One or more chemicals or substances in concentrations in the air high enough to harm humans, animals, vegetation, or materials. Such chemicals or physical conditions (such as excess heat or noise) are called air pollutants.

Albedo   The fraction of the total solar radiation incident on a body that is reflected by it. Albedo can be expressed either as a percentage or a fraction of 1. Snow covered areas have a high albedo (up to about 0.9 or 90%) due to their white colour, while vegetation has a low albedo (generally about 0.1 or 10%) due to the dark colour and light absorbed for photosynthesis. Clouds have an intermediate albedo and are the most important contributor to the Earth's albedo. The Earth's aggregate albedo is approximately 0.3.

Alliance of Small Island States (AOSIS)   The group of Pacific and Caribbean nations who call for relatively fast action by developed nations to reduce greenhouse gas emissions. The AOSIS countries are concerned for the effects of rising sea levels and increased storm activity predicted to accompany global warming.

Alternative energy   Energy derived from non-traditional sources (e.g. compressed natural gas, sun, hydroelectric, wind, geothermal).

Anaerobic decomposition   The breakdown of molecules into simpler molecules or atoms by microorganisms that can survive in partial or complete absence of oxygen.

Antarctic "Ozone Hole"   Refers to the seasonal depletion of stratospheric ozone in a large area over Antarctica.

Anthropogenic   Human made. In the context of greenhouse gases, emissions that are produced as the result of human activities.

Atmosphere   The mixture of gases surrounding the Earth. The Earth's atmosphere consists of about 78.1% nitrogen (by volume), 20.9% oxygen, 0.036% carbon dioxide and trace amounts of other gases. The atmosphere has been divided into a number of imaginary layers according to their mixing or chemical characteristics, generally determined by its thermal properties. The layer nearest to the Earth is the troposphere, which reaches up to an altitude of about 8 km in the polar regions and up to 17 km above the equator. The next is the stratosphere, which reaches to an altitude of about 50 km lies atop the troposphere. The next, mesosphere, extends up to 80-90 km atop the stratosphere, and finally, the thermosphere, or ionosphere, which gradually diminishes and forms a fuzzy border with outer space. See Figure 4 in Chapter 1.

Baseline emissions   The emissions that would occur without policy intervention (in a business-as-usual scenario). Baseline estimates are needed to determine the effectiveness of emissions reduction programs (often called mitigation strategies).

Berlin Mandate   A ruling negotiated at the first *Conference of the Parties* (COP 1), which took place in March, 1995, concluding that the present commitments under the *United Nations Framework Convention on Climate Change* are not adequate. Under the Framework Convention, developed countries pledged to take measures aimed at returning their greenhouse gas emissions to 1990 levels by the year 2000. The Berlin Mandate establishes a process that would enable the Parties to take appropriate action for the period beyond 2000, including strengthening of developed country commitments, through the adoption of a protocol or other legal instruments.

Biodegradable   Material that can be broken down into simpler substances (elements and compounds) by bacteria or other decomposers. Paper and most organic wastes such as animal manure are biodegradable.

Biofuel   Gas or liquid fuel made from plant material (biomass). Includes wood, wood waste, wood liquors, peat, railroad ties, wood sludge, spent sulphite liquors, agricultural waste, straw, tires, fish oils, tall oil, sludge waste, waste alcohol, municipal solid waste, landfill gases, other waste, and ethanol blended into motor gasoline.

Biogeochemical Cycle   Natural processes that recycle nutrients in various chemical forms from the environment, to organisms, and then back to the environment. Examples are the carbon, oxygen, nitrogen, phosphorus, and hydrological cycles.

Biological oxygen demand (BOD)   Amount of dissolved oxygen needed by aerobic decomposers to break down the organic materials in a given volume of water at a certain temperature over a specified time period.

Biomass energy   Energy produced by combusting biomass materials such as wood. The carbon dioxide emitted from burning biomass will not increase total atmospheric carbon dioxide if this consumption is done on a sustainable basis (i.e. if in a given period of time, regrowth of biomass takes up as much carbon dioxide as is released from biomass combustion). Biomass energy is often suggested as a replacement for fossil fuel combustion. See biomass.

Biosphere   The living and dead organisms found near the earth's surface in parts of the lithosphere, atmosphere, and hydrosphere. The part of the global carbon cycle that includes living organisms and biogenic organic matter.

Borehole   Any exploratory hole drilled into the Earth or ice to gather geophysical data. Climate researchers often take *ice core* samples, a type of borehole, to predict atmospheric composition in earlier years. See *ice core*.

Carbon cycle   All carbon reservoirs and exchanges of carbon from reservoir to reservoir by various chemical, physical, geological, and biological processes. Usually thought of as a series of the four main reservoirs of carbon interconnected by pathways of exchange. The four reservoirs, regions of the Earth in which carbon behaves in a systematic manner, are: the atmosphere, terrestrial biosphere (usually includes freshwater systems), oceans, and sediments (includes fossil fuels). Each of these global reservoirs may be subdivided into smaller pools, ranging in size from individual communities or ecosystems to the total of all living organisms (biota).

Carbon dioxide equivalent (CDE)   A metric measure used to compare the emissions from various greenhouse gases based upon their global warming potential (GWP). Carbon dioxide equivalents are commonly expressed as "million metric tons of carbon dioxide equivalents (MMTCDE)." The carbon dioxide equivalent for a gas is derived by multiplying the tons of the gas by the associated GWP.

MMTCDE = (million metric tons of a gas) * (GWP of the gas)

Carbon equivalent (CE)   A metric measure used to compare the emissions of the different greenhouse gases based upon their global warming potential (GWP). Greenhouse gas emissions are most commonly expressed as "million metric tons of carbon equivalents" (MMTCE). Global warming potentials are used to convert greenhouse gases to carbon dioxide equivalents - they can be converted to carbon equivalents by multiplying by 12/44 (the ratio of the molecular weight of carbon to carbon dioxide). The formula for carbon equivalents is:

MMTCE = (million metric tons of a gas) * (GWP of the gas) * (12/44)

Carbon sequestration   The uptake and storage of carbon. Trees and plants, for example, absorb carbon dioxide, release oxygen and store the carbon. Fossil fuels were at one time biomass and continue to store the carbon until burnt.

Carbon sinks   Carbon reservoirs and conditions that take-in and store more carbon (i.e. carbon sequestration) than they release. Carbon sinks can serve to partially offset greenhouse gas emissions. Forests and oceans are large carbon sinks. See *carbon sequestration*.

Chlorofluorocarbons (CFCs)   Organic compounds made up of atoms of carbon, chlorine, and fluorine. An example is CFC-12 ($CCl_{12}F_2$), used as a refrigerant in refrigerators and air conditioners and as a foam blowing agent. Gaseous CFCs can deplete the ozone layer when they slowly rise into the stratosphere, are broken down by strong ultraviolet radiation, release chlorine atoms, and then react with ozone molecules.

Climate   The average weather, usually taken over a 30-year time, for a particular region and time period. Climate is not the same as weather, but rather, it is the average pattern of weather for a particular region. Weather describes the short-term state of the atmosphere. Climatic elements include precipitation, temperature, humidity, sunshine, wind velocity, phenomena such as fog, frost, and hail-storms, and other measures of the weather.

Climate change   The term "climate change" is sometimes used to refer to all forms of climatic inconsistencies, but because the Earth's climate is never static, the term is more properly used to imply a significant change from one climatic condition to another. In some cases, *climate change* has been used synonymously with the term, *global warming*; scientists however, tend to use the term in the wider sense to also include natural changes in climate.

Climate feedback   An atmospheric, oceanic, terrestrial, or other process that is activated by direct climate change induced by changes in radiative forcing. Climate feedbacks may increase (positive feedback) or diminish (negative feedback) the magnitude of the direct climate change.

Climate lag   The delay that occurs in climate change as a result of some factor that changes only very slowly. For example, the effects of releasing more carbon dioxide into the atmosphere may not be known for some time because a large fraction is dissolved in the ocean and only released to the atmosphere many years later.

Climate model   A quantitative way of representing the interactions of the atmosphere, oceans, land surface, and ice. Models can range from relatively simple to quite comprehensive.

Composting   Partial breakdown of organic plant and animal matter by aerobic bacteria to produce a material that can be used as a soil conditioner or fertilizer.

Conference of the Parties (COP)   The supreme body of the United Nations Framework Convention on Climate Change (UNFCCC). It comprises more than 170 nations that have ratified the Convention. Its first session was held in Berlin, Germany, in 1995 and it is expected to continue meeting on a yearly basis. The COP's role is to promote and review the implementation of the Convention. It will periodically review existing commitments in light of the Convention's objective, new scientific findings, and the effectiveness of national climate change programs.

Deforestation Those practices or processes that result in the change of forested lands to non-forest uses. This is often cited as one of the major causes of the enhanced greenhouse effect for two reasons: 1) the burning or decomposition of the wood releases carbon dioxide; and 2) trees that once removed carbon dioxide from the atmosphere in the process of photosynthesis are no longer present and contributing to carbon storage.

Desertification The progressive destruction or degradation of existing vegetative cover to form desert. This can occur due to overgrazing, deforestation, drought, and the burning of extensive areas. Once formed, deserts can only support a sparse range of vegetation. Climatic effects associated with this phenomenon include increased albedo, reduced atmospheric humidity, and greater atmospheric dust (aerosol) loading.

Ecosystem The complex system of plant, animal, fungal, and microorganism communities and their associated non-living environment interacting as an ecological unit. Ecosystems have no fixed boundaries; instead their parameters are set to the scientific, management, or policy questions being examined. Depending upon the purpose of analysis, a single lake, a watershed, or an entire region could be considered an ecosystem.

El Ninõ A climatic phenomenon occurring irregularly, but generally every 3 to 5 years. El Ninõs often first become evident during the Christmas season (El Ninõ means Christ child) in the surface oceans of the eastern tropical Pacific Ocean. The phenomenon involves seasonal changes in the direction of the tropical winds over the Pacific and abnormally warm surface ocean temperatures. The changes in the tropics are most intense in the Pacific region, these changes can disrupt weather patterns throughout the tropics and can extend to higher latitudes, especially in Central and North America. The relationship between these events and global weather patterns are currently the subject of much research in order to enhance prediction of seasonal to interannual fluctuations in the climate.

Emission inventory A list of air pollutants emitted into the atmosphere of a community, state, nation, or the Earth in amounts per some unit time (e.g. day or year) by type of source. An emission inventory has both political and scientific applications.

Emissions The release of a substance (usually a gas when referring to the subject of climate change) into the atmosphere.

Emissions coefficient/factor   A unique value for scaling emissions to activity data in terms of a standard rate of emissions per unit of activity (e.g., grams of carbon dioxide emitted per barrel of fossil fuel consumed).

Enhanced greenhouse effect   The concept that the natural greenhouse effect has been enhanced by anthropogenic emissions of greenhouse gases. Increased concentrations of carbon dioxide, methane, and nitrous oxide, CFCs, HFCs, PFCs, SF6, NF3, and other photochemically important gases caused by human activities such as fossil fuel consumption, trap more infra-red radiation, thereby exerting a warming influence on the climate.

Environment   All external conditions that affect an organism or other specified system during its lifetime.

Fertilization, Carbon dioxide   An expression (sometimes reduced to *fertilization*) used to denote increased plant growth due to a higher carbon dioxide concentration.

Fluorocarbons   Carbon-fluorine compounds that often contain other elements such as hydrogen, chlorine, or bromine. Common fluorocarbons include chlorofluorocarbons (CFCs), hydrochlorofluorocarbons (HCFCs), hydrofluorocarbons (HFCs), and perfluorocarbons (PFCs).

Forcing Mechanism   A process that alters the energy balance of the climate system, i.e. changes the relative balance between incoming solar radiation and outgoing infrared radiation from Earth. Such mechanisms include changes in solar irradiance, volcanic eruptions, and enhancement of the natural greenhouse effect by emission of carbon dioxide.

Fugitive emissions   Unintended gas leaks from the processing, transmission, and/or transportation of fossil fuels, CFCs from refrigeration leaks, SF6 from electrical power distributor, etc.

General Circulation Model (GCM)   A global, three-dimensional computer model of the climate system which can be used to simulate human-induced climate change. GCMs are highly complex and they represent the effects of such factors as reflective and absorptive properties of atmospheric water vapour, greenhouse gas concentrations, clouds, annual and daily solar heating, ocean temperatures and ice boundaries. The most recent GCMs include global representations of the atmosphere, oceans, and land surface.

Global warming   The progressive gradual rise in the earth's surface temperature thought to be caused by the greenhouse effect and responsible for changes in global climate patterns. An increase in the near surface temperature of the Earth. Global warming has occurred in the distant past as the result of natural influences, but the term is most often used to refer to the warming predicted to occur as a result of increased emissions of greenhouse gases.

Global Warming Potential (GWP)   The index used to translate the level of emissions of various gases into a common measure in order to compare the relative radiative forcing of different gases without directly calculating the changes in atmospheric concentrations. GWPs are calculated as the ratio of the radiative forcing that would result from the emissions of one kilogram of a greenhouse gas to that from emission of one kilogram of carbon dioxide over a period of time (usually 100 years).

Greenhouse effect   The effect produced as greenhouse gases allow incoming solar radiation to pass through the Earth's atmosphere, but prevent part of the outgoing infrared radiation from the Earth's surface and lower atmosphere from escaping into outer space. This process occurs naturally and has kept the Earth's temperature about 59 degrees F warmer than it would otherwise be. Current life on Earth could not be sustained without the natural greenhouse effect.

Greenhouse gas   Any gas that absorbs infra-red radiation in the atmosphere. Greenhouse gases include water vapor, carbon dioxide, methane, nitrous oxide, halogenated fluorocarbons (HCFCs), ozone (O_3), perfluorinated carbons (PFCs), and hydrofluorocarbons (HFCs).

Hydrochlorofluorocarbons (HCFCs)   Compounds containing hydrogen, fluorine, chlorine, and carbon atoms. Although ozone depleting substances, they are less potent at destroying stratospheric ozone than chlorofluorocarbons (CFCs). They have been introduced as temporary replacements for CFCs and are also greenhouse gases. See *ozone depleting substance.*

Hydrofluorocarbons (HFCs)   Compounds containing hydrogen, fluorine, and carbon atoms only. They were introduced as alternatives to ozone depleting substances in serving many industrial, commercial, and personal needs. HFCs are emitted as by-products of industrial processes and are also used in manufacturing. They do not significantly deplete the stratospheric ozone layer, but they are powerful greenhouse gases with global warming potentials ranging from 140 (HFC-152a) to 11,700 (HFC-23).

Hydrologic cycle   The process of evaporation, vertical and horizontal transport of vapor, condensation, precipitation, and the flow of water from continents to oceans. It is a major factor in determining climate through its influence on surface vegetation, the clouds, snow and ice, and soil moisture. The hydrologic cycle is responsible for 25 to 30 percent of the mid-latitudes' heat transport from the equatorial to polar regions.

Infrared radiation   The heat energy that is emitted from all solids, liquids, and gases. In the context of the greenhouse issue, the term refers to the heat energy emitted by the Earth's surface and its atmosphere. Greenhouse gases strongly absorb this radiation in the Earth's atmosphere, and radiate some back towards the surface, creating the greenhouse effect.

Intergovernmental Panel on Climate Change (IPCC)   The IPCC was established jointly by the United Nations Environment Programme and the World Meteorological Organization in 1988. The aim of the IPCC is to assess information in the scientific and technical literature related to all significant components of the issue of climate change. The IPCC draws upon hundreds of the world's expert scientists as authors and thousands as expert reviewers. Leading experts on climate change and environmental, social, and economic sciences from some 60 nations help the IPCC preparing periodic assessments of the scientific underpinnings for understanding global climate change and its consequences. With its capacity for reporting on climate change, its consequences, and the viability of adaptation and mitigation measures, the IPCC is also considered as the official advisory body to the world's governments on the state of the science of the climate change issue. For example, the IPCC organized the development of internationally accepted methods for conducting national greenhouse gas emission inventories.

Joint implementation   Agreements made between two or more nations under the auspices of the *United Nations Framework Convention on Climate Change* to help reduce greenhouse gas emissions.

Kyoto Protocol   This is an international agreement struck by 159 nations attending the Third Conference of Parties (COP) to the United Nations Framework Convention on Climate Change (held in December 1997 in Kyoto Japan) to reduce worldwide emissions of greenhouse gases. If ratified and put into force, individual countries have committed to reduce their greenhouse gas emissions by a specified amount.

Landfill Land waste disposal site in which waste is generally spread in thin layers, compacted, and covered with a fresh layer of soil each day.

Lifetime (Atmospheric) The lifetime of a greenhouse gas refers to the approximate amount of time it would take for the anthropogenic increment to an atmospheric pollutant concentration to return to its natural level (assuming emissions cease) as a result of either being converted to another chemical compound or being taken out of the atmosphere via a sink. This time depends on the pollutant's sources and sinks as well as its reactivity. The lifetime of a pollutant is often considered in conjunction with the mixing of pollutants in the atmosphere; a long lifetime will allow the pollutant to mix throughout the atmosphere. Average lifetimes can vary from about a week (sulphate aerosols) to more than a century (CFCs, carbon dioxide).

Long-wave radiation The radiation emitted in the spectral wavelength greater than 4 micrometers corresponding to the radiation emitted from the Earth and atmosphere. It is sometimes referred to as terrestrial radiation or infrared radiation, although somewhat imprecisely.

Methane (CH_4) A hydrocarbon that is a greenhouse gas with a global warming potential most recently estimated at 21. Methane is produced through anaerobic (without oxygen) decomposition of waste in landfills, animal digestion, decomposition of animal wastes, production and distribution of natural gas and petroleum, coal production, and incomplete fossil fuel combustion.

Methanotrophic Having the biological capacity to oxidize methane to CO_2 and water by metabolism under aerobic conditions.

Montreal Protocol (on Substances that Deplete the Ozone Layer) The Montreal Protocol and its amendments control the phaseout of ozone depleting substances, their production and use. Under the Protocol, several international organizations report on the science of ozone depletion, implement projects to help move away from ozone depleting substances, and provide a forum for policy discussions. In the United States, the Protocol is implemented under the Clean Air Act Amendments of 1990.

Mount Pinatubo A volcano in the Philippine Islands that erupted in 1991. The eruption of Mount Pinatubo ejected enough particulate and sulphate aerosol matter into the atmosphere to block some of the incoming solar radiation from reaching Earth's atmosphere.

This effectively cooled the planet from 1992 to 1994, masking the warming that had been occurring for most of the 1980s and 1990s.

Natural gas   Underground deposits of gases consisting of 50 to 90 per cent methane (CH_4) and small amounts of heavier gaseous hydrocarbon compounds such as propane (C_3H_4) and butane (C_4H_{10}).

Nitrogen cycle   Cyclic movement of nitrogen in different chemical forms from the environment, to organisms, and then back to the environment.

Nitrogen oxides (NOx)   Gases consisting of one molecule of nitrogen and varying numbers of oxygen molecules. Nitrogen oxides are produced, for example, by the combustion of fossil fuels in vehicles and electric power plants. In the atmosphere, nitrogen oxides can contribute to formation of photochemical ozone (smog), impair visibility, and have health consequences; they are considered pollutants.

Nitrous oxide (N_2O)   A powerful greenhouse gas with a global warming potential most recently evaluated at 310. Major sources of nitrous oxide include soil cultivation practices, especially the use of commercial and organic fertilizers, fossil fuel combustion, nitric acid production, and biomass burning.

Ozone (O_3)   A colorless gas with a pungent odor, having the molecular form of O3 , found in two layers of the atmosphere, the stratosphere (about 90% of the total atmospheric loading) and the troposphere (about 10%). Ozone is a form of oxygen found naturally in the stratosphere that provides a protective layer shielding the Earth from ultraviolet radiation's harmful health effects on humans and the environment. In the troposphere, ozone is a chemical oxidant and major component of photochemical smog. Ozone can seriously affect the human respiratory system.

Ozone depleting substance (ODS)   A family of man-made compounds that includes, but are not limited to, chlorofluorocarbons (CFCs), bromofluorocarbons (halons), methyl chloroform, carbon tetrachloride, methyl bromide, and hydrochlorofluorocarbons (HCFCs). These compounds have been shown to deplete stratospheric ozone, and therefore are typically referred to as ODSs.

Ozone layer   The layer of gaseous ozone (O_3) in the stratosphere that protects life on earth by filtering out harmful ultraviolet radiation from the sun.

Ozone precursors   Chemical compounds, such as carbon monoxide, methane, non-methane hydrocarbons, and nitrogen oxides, which in the presence of solar radiation react with other chemical compounds to form ozone, mainly in the troposphere.

Perfluorocarbons (PFCs)   A group of human-made chemicals composed of carbon and fluorine only. These chemicals (predominantly CF_4 and C_2F_6) were introduced as alternatives, along with hydrofluorocarbons, to the ozone depleting substances. In addition, PFCs are emitted as by-products of industrial processes and are also used in manufacturing. PFCs do not harm the stratospheric ozone layer, but they are powerful greenhouse gases: CF_4 has a global warming potential (GWP) of 6,500 and C_2F_6 has a GWP of 9,200.

Pollution   A change in the physical, chemical, or biological characteristics of the air, water, or soil that can affect the health, survival, or activities of humans in an unwanted way. Some expand the term to include harmful effects on all forms of life.

Radiative forcing   A change in the balance between incoming solar radiation and outgoing infrared radiation. Without any radiative forcing, solar radiation coming to the Earth would continue to be approximately equal to the infrared radiation emitted from the Earth. The addition of greenhouse gases traps an increased fraction of the infrared radiation, radiating it back toward the surface and creating a warming influence (i.e., positive radiative forcing because incoming solar radiation will exceed outgoing infrared radiation).

Recycling   Collecting and reprocessing a resource so it can be used again. An example is collecting aluminum cans, melting them down, and using the aluminum to make new cans or other aluminum products.

Renewable energy   Energy obtained from sources that are essentially inexhaustible, unlike, for example, the fossil fuels, of which there is a finite supply. Renewable sources of energy include wood, waste, geothermal, wind, photovoltaic, and solar thermal energy.

Residence time   The average time spent in a reservoir by an individual atom or molecule. With respect to greenhouse gases, residence time usually refers to how long a particular molecule remains in the atmosphere.

Sink   A reservoir that uptakes a chemical element or compound from another part of its cycle. For example, soil and trees tend to act as natural sinks for carbon.

Stratosphere   Second layer of the atmosphere, extending from about 19 to 48 kilometers (12 to 30 miles) above the earth's surface. It contains small amounts of gaseous ozone (O_3), which filters out about 99 percent of the incoming harmful ultraviolet (UV) radiation. Most commercial airline flights operate at a cruising altitude in the lower stratosphere.

Sulphate aerosols   Particulate matter that consists of compounds of sulphur formed by the interaction of sulphur dioxide and sulphur trioxide with other compounds in the atmosphere. Sulphate aerosols are injected into the atmosphere from the combustion of fossil fuels and the eruption of volcanoes like Mt. Pinatubo. Recent theory suggests that sulphate aerosols may lower the earth's temperature by reflecting away solar radiation (negative radiative forcing). General Circulation Models which incorporate the effects of sulphate aerosols more accurately predict global temperature variations.

Synthetic natural gas (SNG)   A manufactured product chemically similar in most respects to natural gas, resulting from the conversion or reforming of petroleum hydrocarbons. It may easily be substituted for, or interchanged with, pipeline quality natural gas.

Terrestrial radiation   The total infrared radiation emitted by the Earth and its atmosphere in the temperature range of approximately 200 to 300 ^{O}K. Terrestrial radiation provides a major part of the potential energy changes necessary to drive the atmospheric wind system and is responsible for maintaining the surface air temperature within limits of livability.

Trace Gas   Any one of the less common gases found in the Earth's atmosphere. Nitrogen, oxygen, and argon make up more than 99 percent of the Earth's atmosphere. Other gases, such as carbon dioxide, water vapor, methane, oxides of nitrogen, ozone, and ammonia, are considered trace gases. Although relatively unimportant in terms of their absolute volume, they have significant effects on the Earth's weather and climate.

Troposphere   The lowest layer of the atmosphere and contains about 95 percent of the mass of air in the Earth's atmosphere. The troposphere extends from the Earth's surface up to about 10 to 15 kilometers. All weather processes take place in the troposphere. Ozone that is formed in the troposphere plays a significant role in both the greenhouse gas effect and urban smog.

Ultraviolet radiation (UV)   A portion of the electromagnetic spectrum with wavelengths shorter than visible light. The sun produces UV, which is commonly split into three bands of decreasing wavelength. Shorter wavelength radiation has a greater potential to cause biological damage on living organisms. The longer wavelength ultraviolet band, UVA, is not absorbed by ozone in the atmosphere. UVB is mostly absorbed by ozone, although some reaches the Earth. The shortest wavelength band, UVC, is completely absorbed by ozone and normal oxygen in the atmosphere.

United Nations Framework Convention on Climate Change (UNFCCC) The international treaty unveiled at the United Nations Conference on Environment and Development (UNCED) in June 1992. The UNFCCC commits signatory countries to stabilize anthropogenic (i.e. human-induced) greenhouse gas emissions to "levels that would prevent dangerous anthropogenic interference with the climate system." The UNFCCC also requires that all signatory parties develop and update national inventories of anthropogenic emissions of all greenhouse gases not otherwise controlled by the Montreal Protocol. Out of 155 countries that have ratified this accord, the United States was the first industrialized nation to do so.

Water Vapours It is the water present in the atmosphere in gaseous form. Water vapor is an important part of the natural greenhouse effect. While humans are not significantly increasing its concentration, it contributes to the enhanced greenhouse effect because the warming influence of greenhouse gases leads to a positive water vapour feedback. In addition to its role as a natural greenhouse gas, water vapour plays an important role in regulating the temperature of the planet because clouds form when excess water vapour in the atmosphere condenses to form ice and water droplets and precipitation.

Weather Weather is the specific condition of the atmosphere at a particular place and time. It is measured in terms of such constituents as wind, temperature, humidity, atmospheric pressure, cloudiness, and precipitation. In most places, weather can change from hour-to-hour, day-to-day, and season-to-season. Climate is the average weather over a time period and space.

Bibiliography

Adams, R.M., Flemming, R.A., Chang, C.C., McCarl, B.A. and Rosenzweig, C. (1995) A reassessment of the economic effects of global climate change on U.S. agriculture. Climatic Change 30: 147-167.

Adamsen, A.P.S. and King, G.M. (1993) Methane consumption in temperate and sub-arctic forest soils: Rates, vertical zonation and responses to water and nitrogen. Appl. Environ. Microbiol. 59: 485-490.

Adhya, T.K., Patnaik, P., Satpathy, S.N., Kumaraswamy, S. and Sethunathan, N. (1998) Influence of phosphorous application on methane emission and production in flooded paddy soils. Soil Biol. Biochem. 30: 177-181.

Aggarwal, P.K. and Kalra, N. (1994) Analyzing the limitations set by climatic factors, genotype, and water and nitrogen availability on productivity of wheat. II. Climatically potential yields and optimal management strategies. Field Crops Res. 38: 93-103.

Aggarwal, P.K., Kalra, N. and Sankaran, V.M. (1998) Modelling the growth and yield potential of Wheat.in Nagarajan, S., Singh, G. and Tyagi B.S. (Eds). *Wheat research needs beyond 2000 AD*. Proceedings of the international group meetings on "Wheat Research Needs beyond 2000AD". Held at Directorate of wheat research, Karnal, India during 12-14 August, 1997.

Anderson, I.C., Levine, J.S., Poth, M.A. and Riggan, P.J. (1988) Enhanced bionic emissions of nitric oxide and nitrous oxide following surface biomes burning. J. Geophys. Res. 93: 3893-3898.

Arah, J.R.M. (1988) Modeling denitrification in aggregated structureless soils. In: Jenkinson, D.S. and Smith, K.A. (eds.), Nitrogen efficiency in Agricultural Soils, Elsinier, London, pp. 433-444.

Arah, J.R.M. and Smith, K.A. (1989) Steady state denitrification in aggregated soils: a mathematical model. J. Soil Sci. 40: 139-149.

Aulakh, M. S. and Doran, J. W. (2002) Impacts of integrated management of crop residues, green manure and fertilizer N on productivity, C sequestration, denitrification and N_2O emissions in rice-wheat system.17th WCSS, 10th Symposium: Paper no. 9.

Aulakh, M.S., Doran, J.W. and Mosier, A.R. (1992) Soil denitrification—significance, measurement, and effects of management. Adv. Soil Sci. 18: 2-42.

Aulakh, M.S., Wassmann, R. and Rennenberg, H. (2001) Methane emissions from rice fields- Quantification, mechanisms, role of management and mitigation option. Adv. Agron. 70: 193-260.

Baker, J.T. and Allen, L.H. (1993) Effects of CO_2 and the temperature on rice. A summary of five growing regions. J. Agric. Meteorol. 48(5): 575-582.

Baladioli, M., Engel, T., Klocking, B., Priesack, E., Schaaf, T., Sperr, C. and Wang, E. (1994) xpert-N, ein Baukasten zur Simulation der Stickstoffdynamik in Boden und Pflanze. Prototyp, benutzerhandbuch, Lehreinheit fur Ackerbau und Informatik im Pflanzenbau, TU Munchen, Freising, 1-106 (in German).

Banerjee, B., Pathak, H., and Aggarwal, P.K. (2002) Effects of dicyandiamide, farmyard manure and irrigation on ammonia volatilization from an alluvial soil in rice (*Oryza sativa* L.)-wheat (*Triticum aestivum* L.) cropping system. Biol. Fertil. Soils. 36:207-214.

Banerjee, N.K. and Mosier, A.R. (1989) Coated calcium carbide as a nitrification inhibitor in upland and flooded soils. J. Ind. Soc. Soil Sci. 37: 306-313.

Batjes, N.H. (1998) Mitigation of atmospheric CO_2 concentration by increased carbon sequestration in the soil. Biol. Fert. Soil 27(3): 230-235.

Battle, M., Bender, M., Sowers, T., Tans, P.P., Butler, J.H., Elkins, J.W., Ellis, J.T., Conway, T., Zhang, N., Lang, P. and Clarke, A.D. (1996) Atmospheric gas concentrations over the past century measured in air from fin at the south pole. Nature 383: 231-235.

Bhattacharya, S. and Mitra, A.P. (1998) Greenhouse gas emissions in India for the base year 1990. Scientific report No. 11. National Physical Laboratory, New Delhi.

Blake, D.R., Mayer, E.W., Tyler, S.C., Makide, Y., Montague, D.C. and Rowland, F.S. (1982) Global increase in atmospheric methane concentration between 1978 and 1980. Geophys. Res. Lett. 9: 477-480.

Bremner, J.M. and Blackmer, A.M. (1979) Effects of acetylene and soil water content on emissions of nitrous oxide from soils. Nature 280: 380-381.

Bundy, L.G. and Bremmer, J.H. (1974) Effects of nitrification inhibitors on transformation of urea nitrogen in soil. Soil Biol. Biochem. 6: 369-376.

Buresh, R.J., Woodhead, T., Shepherd, K.D., Flordelis, E. and Cabangon, R.C. (1989) Nitrate accumulation and loss in a mung bean-lowland rice cropping system. Soil Sci. Soc. Am. J. 53: 477-482.

Burton, D.L. and Beauchamp, E.G. (1985) Denitrification rate relationships with soil parameters in the field. Commun. Soil. Sci. Plant Anal. 16: 539-549.

Buyanovsky, G.A., Wagner, G.H. and Gantzer, C.J. (1986) Soil respiration in a winter wheat ecosystem. Soil Sci. Soc. Am. J. 50: 338-344.

Cai, Z.C., Xing, G.X., Shen,G.Y., Xu, H., Yuan, Yan, X., Tsuruta, H., Yagi, K. and Minami, K. (1997) Measurement of methane and nitrous oxide emissions from rice paddies in Fengqui, China. Soil. Sci. Plant Nutr. 45(1): 1-13.

Campbell, C. A., McConkey, B. G., Zenter, R. P., Dyck, F. B., Selles, F. and Curtin, D. (1995) Carbon sequestration in a Brown Chernozem as affected by tillage and rotation. Canadain J. Soil Sci. 75: 449-458.

Castaldi, S. and Smith, K.A. (1998) Effect of cyclohexamide on N_2O and NO_3-production in a forest and an agricultural soil. Biol. Fertil. Soils 27: 27-34.

Chaareonsi, N., Budhaboon, C., Pronmart, P. and Wassmann, R. (2000) Methane emission from Deep water rice fields in Thailand. Nutr. Cycl. Agroecosys. 58: 121-130.

Chander, K., Goyal, S., Mundra, M. C. and Kapoor, K. K. (1997) Organic matter, microbial biomass and enzyme activity of soils under different crop rotations in the tropics. Bio. Fert. Soils 24: 306-310.

Chatterjee, A. (1998) Simulating the impact of increase in Carbon Dioxide and temperature on growth and yield of Maize and Sorghum. M.Sc. thesis, Division of Environmental Sciences, Indian Agricultural Research Institute, New Delhi.

Chattopadhayay, R. (2000) Simulating the impact of climatic variability and climate change on the productivity of sugarcane. Ph.D. Thesis, Division of Environmental Sciences, Indian Agricultural Research Institute, New Delhi.

Cicerone, R.J. and Shetter, J.D. (1981) Sources of atmospheric methane: measurements in rice paddies and a discussion. J. Geophys. Res. 86: 7203-7209.

Cohen, S., Wheaton, E. and Masterton, J. (1992) Impacts of climatic change scenarios in the prairie provinces: A case study from Canada. SRC Publication No. E-2900-4-D-92. Saskatchewan Research Council, Saskatoon, Canada.

Conrad, R. (1995) Soil microbial processes involved in production and consumption of atmospheric trace gases. Adv. Microbial Ecol. 14: 207-250.

Dadhwal, V.K. and Nayak, S.R. (1993) A preliminary estimate of biogeochemical cycle of carbon for India. Sci. Cult. 59(1-2): 9-13.

Davidson, E.A. (1992) Sources of nitric oxide and nitrous oxide following wetting of dry soil. Soil Sci. Soc. Am. J. 56: 95-102.

De Datta, S.K. and Buresh, R.J. (1989) Integrated N management in irrigated rice. Adv. Agron. 10: 143-169.

Debnath, G., Jain, M.C., Kumar, S., Sarkar, K. and Sinha, S.K. (1996) Methane emissions from rice fields amended with biogas slurry and farm yard manure. Climatic Change 33: 97-109.

Donner, L. and Ramanathan, V. (1980) Methane and nitrous oxide: their effects on the terrestrial climate. J Atoms. Sci. 37, 119-124.

Duxbury, J. M., Bouldin, D.R., Terry, R.E. and Tate, R.L. III. (1982) Emissions of nitrous oxide from soils. Nature 275: 602-604.

Duxbury, J.M. and McConnaughey, P.K. (1986) Effect of fertilizer source on denitrification and nitrous oxide emissions in a maize-field. Soil Sci. Soc. Am. J. 50: 644-648.

Ehhalt, D.H. (1978) The CH_4 concentration over the ocean and it possible variation with latitude. Tellus 30: 169-176.

Ehhalt, D.H. and Heidt, L.E. (1973) Vertical profiles of CH_4 in the troposphere and Stratosphere. J. Geophys. Res. 78: 5265-5271.

Eichner, M.J. (1990) Nitrous oxide emission from fertilized soils: Summary of avialable data. J. Environ. Qual. 19: 272-280.

Etheridge, D. M., Steele, L. P., Langenfields, R. I., Francey, R. J., Bamola, I. M. and Morgan, V. I. (1996) Natural and anthropogenic changes in atmospheric CO_2 over the last 1000 years from aim in Antarctic ice and fem. J. Geophys. Res. 101: 4115-4128.

FAO. (2000) Carbon Sequestration Options Under the Clean Development Mechanism to Address Land Degradation. World Soil Resources Reports 92. FAO and IFAD, Rome

Fenn, L.B. and Hossner, L.R. (1985) Ammonia volatilization from ammonium as ammonium forming nitrogen fertilizers. Adv. Soil Sci. 1: 123-169.

Ferm, M. (1998) Atmospheric ammonia and ammonium transport in Europe and critical loads: a review. Nutr. Cycl. Agroecosys. 51: 5-17.

Fillery, I.R.P. and Vlek, P.L.G. (1986) Reappraisal of the significance of ammonia volatilization as N-loss mechanism in flooded rice fields. Fert. Res. 9: 79-98.

Fillery, I.R.P., Roger, P.A. and De Datta, S.K. (1986) Ammonia volatilization from nitrogen sources applied to rice-fields. II. Floodwater properties and submerged photosynthetic biomass. Soil Sci. Soc. Am. J. 50: 86-91.

Fillery, I.R.P., Simpson, J.R. and De Datta, S.K. (1984) Influence of field environment and fertilizer management on ammonia loss from flooded rice. Soil Sci. Soc. Am. J. 48: 914-920.

Firestone M. K. and Davidson E. A. (1989) Microbiological basis of NO and N_2O prod. and consumption in soil In : Andreae M. O. and Schimel D. S. (Eds) Exchange of trace gases between terrestrial ecosystem and the Atmosphere, John Willy and Sons Ltd. Chichester, UK. 7-21pp.

Fisher, G. and Heilig, G. K. (1997) Population momentum and demand on land and water resources. Phil. Trans. Royal Soc. (London) Ser. B. 352: 869-889.

Galbally, I.E. (1985) In: The biogeochemical cycling of sulfur and nitrogen in the remote atmosphere. Galloway *et al.* (Eds) D. Reidel Publication Co. Boston, MA.

Garg, A. and Shukla, P.R. (2002) Emission inventory of India. Tata McGraw-Hill Publishing Co., New Delhi 278 p.

Gebhart, D.L., Johnson, H.B., Mayeux, H. S. and Polley, H. W. (1994) The CRP increases soil organic carbon. J. Soil and Water Cons. 49: 488-492.

George, T., Ladha, J.K., Buresh, R.J. and Garrity, D.P. (1992) Managing native and legume fixed N in lowland rice based cropping systems. Plant Soil 141: 69-91.

Gorissen, A., Van Ginkel, J.H., Keurentjes, J.J.B. and Van Veen, J.A. (1995) Grass root decomposition is retarded when grass has been grown under elevated CO_2. Soil Biol. Biochem. 27: 117-120.

Granli, T. and Bockman, O.C. (1994) Nitrous oxide from agriculture. Norwegian J. Agri. Sci. 12: 128-134.

Gupta, P.K. and Mitra, A.P. (1999) Greenhouse gas emissions in India. ADB-Methane Asia Campaign (MAC) Scientific report No. 19. National Physical Laboratory, New Delhi.

Gupta, Raj K. and Rao, D.L.N. (1994) Potential of wastelands for sequestering carbon by reforestation. Curr. Sci. 66(5):73-75.

Hargrove, W.L., Rock, B.R., Raunikar, R.A. and Urban, W.J. (1987) Comparison of a forced-draft technique to ^{15}N recovery for measuring ammonia volatilization under field conditions. Soil Sci. Soc. Am. J. 51: 124-128.

Holzapfel- Pschorn, A. and Seiler, W. (1986) Methane emission during a cultivation period from an Italian rice paddy. J. Geophys. Res. 91: 11803-11814.

Houghton, R.A. (1995) Emission of carbon from land-use change. In T.M.L. Wigley and D.S. Schimel (Eds). Carbon cycle. Cambridge University Press, Stanford, CT.

Hrtwig, U.A., Zanetti, S., Hebeisen, T., Luscher, A.,Frehner, M., Fischer, B., van Kessel, C., Hendrey,G.R., Blum, H and Nosberger, J. (1996) Symbiotic nitrogen fixation: one key to understand the response of temperate grasslands to ecosystems to elevated CO_2? Korner, C. and Bazzaz, F.A., Eds, In Community, population, and evolutionary responses to elevated CO_2 concentration, Academic Press, New York. 253-264 pp.

Huggins, D.R., Allan, D. L., Gardener, J. C., Karlen, D. L., Bezdicek, D. F., Rosek, M. J. Alms, Flock, M., Miller, B. S. and Staben, M. L. (1997) Enhancing carbon sequestration in CRP-managed land In: R. Lal, J. Kimble, R. F. Follett and B. A. Stewart (Eds.) Soil Processes and the carbon cycle. CRC Press LLC. Boca Raton. pp. 323-334.

Hulme, M., Wigley, T., Jiang, T., Zhao, Z., Wang, F., Ding, Y., Leemans, R. and Markham, A. (1992). Climate Change due to the Greenhouse Effect and its Implications for China. CRU/WWF/SMA, World Wide Fund for Nature, Gland, Switzerland.

Hume, C.J., and Cattle, H. (1990) The greenhouse effect: meteorological mechanisms and methods. Outlook Agric. 19: 17-23.

Hutchinson, G.L., and Mosier, A.R. (1981) Improved soil cover method for field measurement of nitrous oxide flux. Soil Sci. Soc. Am. J. 45: 311-316.

Hutsch, B.W. (1998) Methane oxidation in arable soil as inhibited by ammonium, nitrite, and organic manure with respect to soil pH. Biol. Fertil. Soils 28: 27-35.

IPCC (1990) Intergovernmental Panel on Climate Change. In: Houghton, J.T., Jenkins, G.T. and Ephraums, J.T. (Eds.) The IPCC Scientific Assessment in Cambridge University Press, Cambridge.

IPCC (1996) Climate Change (1995), Impacts, adaptations and mitigation of climate change. Scientific Technical Report Analyses. Contribution of Working Group II to the Second Assessment Report of the Intergovernmental Panel on Climate Change. Watson, R.T., Zinyowera, M.C. and Ross, R.H. (Eds), Cambridge and New York, p. 880.

IRRI (1995) World rice statistics, 1993-94, International Rice Research Institute, Manila, Philippines.

Jain, M.C., Kumar, S., Wassmann, R., Mitra, S., Singh, S.D., Singh, J.P., Singh, R., Yadav, A.K. and Gupta, S. (2000) Methane emissions from irrigated rice fields in northern India (New Delhi). Nutr. Cycl. Agroecosys. 58: 75-83.

Johnson, D.E. Phetteplace, H.W. and Seidl, A.F. (2001). Methane, nitrous oxide and carbon dioxide emissions from ruminant livestock production systems. Proc. 1stInter. Conf. Greenhouse Gases and Animal Agric., Obihiro, Japan. Nov. 2001.

Kicklighter, D.W., Melillo, J.M., Peterjohn, W.T., Rastetter, E.B., McGuire, A.D. and Steudler, P.A. (1994) Aspects of spatial and temporal aggregation in estimating regional carbon dioxide fluxes from temperate forest soils. J. Geophys. Res. 99: 1303-1315.

Kumar, U, Jain, M.C., Kumar, S., Pathak, H. and Majumdar, D. (2000) Role of nitrification inhibitors on nitrous oxide emissions in a fertilized alluvial clay loam under different moisture regimes. Curr. Sci. 79: 224-228.

Ladha, J.K., Fischer, K.S., Hossain, M., Hobbs, P.R. and Hardy, B. (2000) Improving the productivity and sustainability of rice-wheat systems of the Indo-Gangetic Plains: a synthesis of NARS-IRRI partnership research, Discussion Paper No. 40. International Rice Research Institute, Philippines, p 31.

Lal, R. (1997) Degradation and resilience of soils. Phil. Trans. Roy. Soc. B. 352: 997-1010.

Lal, R. (2001) World crop land soils as a source or sink for atmospheric carbon. Adv. Agro. 71: 145-191.

Lal, R., Follett, R. F., Kimble, J. and Cole, C. V. (1999) Managing US cropland to sequester carbon in soil. J. Soil Water Cons. 54: 374-381.

Lal, R., Kimble, J. and Steward, B.A. (1995) In: Eds Lal, R., Kimble, J., Levine, E. and

Steward, B.A. *Soil Management and Greenhouse Effect* Lewis Publishers, London, 373-385.

Lamb, J.A., Peterson, G.A. and Fenster, C.R. (1985) Wheat fallow tillage systems effect on a newly cultivated grassland soils nitrogen budget. Soil Sci. Soc. Am. J. 49: 352-354.

Lessard, R.; Rochette, P., Topp, E., Pattey, E., Desjardins, R.L. and Beaumont, G. (1994) Methane and carbon dioxide fluxes from poorly drained adjacent cultivated and forest sites. Canadian J. Soil Sci. 74: 139-148.

Li, C. S. (2000) Modelling trace gas emissions from agricultural ecosystems. Nutr. Cycling Agroecosys. 58: 259-276.

Lu, W.F., Chen, W. Duan, B.W., Guo, W. M., Lu, Y., Lantin, R.S., Wassmann, R. and Neue, H.U. (2000) Methane emission and mitigation options in irrigated rice fields in southeast China. Nutr. Cycling. Agroecosys. 58: 65-74.

Machida, T., Nakazawa, T., Fujii Yaola, S. and Watanabe, O. (1995) Increase in the atmospheric nitrous oxide concentration during the last 250 years. Geophys. Res. Lett. 22: 2921-2924.

Majumdar, D., Dutta, A. Kumar, S., Pathak, H., and Jain, M.C. (2001) Mitigation of N_2O emission from an alluvial soil by application of karanjin. Biol. Fertil. Soils 33: 438-442.

Majumdar, D., Kumar, S., Pathak, H., Jain, M.C. and Kumar, U. (2000) Reducing nitrous oxide emission from rice field with nitrification inhibitors. Agric. Ecosys. Environ. 81: 163-169.

Migeotte, M.V. (1948) Spectroscopic evidence of methane in the earth's atmosphere. Phys. Rev. 73: 519-520.

Mishra, S., Rath, A. K., Adhya, T.K., Rao, V.R. and Sethunathan, N. (1997) Effect of continuous flooding and alternate water regimes on methane efflux from rice under greenhouse conditions. Biol. Fertil. Soils 24: 399-407.

Mitsch, W. J. and Wu, X. (1995) Wetlands and global change In: R. Lal, J. Kimble, E. Levine and B. A. Stewart (Eds) Soil management and greenhouse effect, CRC / Lewis Publishers Boca Raton. FL, 205-230.

More, S.D. and Varade, S.B. (1978) Volatilization losses of ammonia from different nitrogen carriers as affected by soil moisture, organic matter and method of fertilizer application. J. Indian Soc. Soil Sci. 26(2): 112-115.

Mosier, A., Schimel, D., Valentine, D., Bronson, K. and Parton, W. (1991) Methane and nitrous oxide fluxes in native, fertilized and cultivated grasslands. Nature 350: 330.

Mosier, A.R., (1998) Soil process and global change. Biol. Fertil. Soils 27: 221-229.

Mosier, A.R., Duxbury, J.M., Freney, J.R., Heinemeyer, O. and Minami, K. (1996) Nitrous oxide emissions from agricultural fields: Assessment, measurement and mitigation. Plant Soil 181: 95-108.

Mosier, A.R., Duxbury, J.M., Freney, J.R., Heinemeyer, O. and Minami, K. (1998) Assessing and mitigating N_2O emissions from agricultural soils. Climatic Change 40: 7-38.

Neue, H. U. (1997) Fluxes of methane from rice fields and potential for mitigation. Soil Use Manage. 13: 258-267.

Neue, H.U., Wassmann, R., Kludze, H.K., Wang, B. and Lantin, R.L. (1997) Factors and processes controlling methane emissions from rice fields. Nutr. Cycling Agroecosys. 49: 111-117.

Oremland, R.M. (1988) Biogeochemistry of methanogenic bacteria. In: Biology of anaerobic microorganisms (Ed. Zehnder A J B). John Wiley Sons, New York, pp. 641-706.

Page, A.L., Miller, R.H. and Keeney, D.R. (1982) Methods of soil analysis. Part 2, Chemical and microbiological properties, 2nd edition, Agronomy No. 9, ASA-SSSA, Madison, WI, USA, p 1159.

Palmer, R.R. and Reeve, J.N. (1993) Methanogen gene and molecular biology of methane biosynthesis. In Genetics and Molecular Biology of Anaerobic Bacteria. (Ed. Sebald, M.), Springer-Verlag, Berlin, Germany, 13-35 pp.

Parashar, D.C., Kulshreshtha, U.C. and Sharma, C. (1998) Anthropogenic missions of NOx, NH3 and N2O in India. Nutr. Cycling Agroecosys. 52: 255-259.

Parkin, T.B. (1987) Soil microsites as a source of denitrification variability. Soil Sci. Soc. Am. J. 51: 1194-1199.

Parton, W.J., Mosier, A.R., Ojima, D.S., Valentine, D.W, Schimel, D.S., Weier, K. and Kulmala, A.E. (1996) Generalized models for N2 and N2O production from nitrification and denitrification. Global Biogeochem. Cycles 10(3): 401-412.

Pathak, H. (1999) Emissions of nitrous oxide from soil. Curr. Sci. 77: 359-369.

Pathak, H. and Banerjee, B. (2003) Ammonia emission from soil: Environmental consequences, mechanisms, factors and mitigation options. Fert. News (submitted).

Pathak, H. and Nedwell, D.B. (2001) Strategies to reduce nitrous oxide emission from soil with fertiliser selection and nitrification inhibitor. Water Air Soil Pollution 129: 217-228.

Pathak, H. and Rao, D.L.N. (1998) Carbon and nitrogen mineralization from added organic matter in saline and alkali soils. Soil Biol. Biochem. 30(6): 695-702.

Pathak, H., Bhatia, A., Shiv Prasad, Jain, M.C., Kumar, S., Singh, S. and Kumar, U. (2002) Emission of nitrous oxide from soil in rice-wheat systems of Indo-Gangetic plains of India. J. Environ. Monit. Assess. 77(2): 163-178.

Pathak, H., Dwivedi, M.K., Sharma, S.K. Harit, R.C. and Singh, P. (1998) Effect of some chemicals on N-use efficiency in maize-wheat cropping system. Fert. News 43(11): 53-57.

Pathak, H., Ladha, J.K., Aggarwal, P.K., Peng, S., Das, S., Yadvinder Singh, Bijay-Singh, Kamra, S.K., Mishra, B., Sastri, A.S.R.A.S., Aggarwal, H.P., Das D.K. and Gupta, R.K. (2003a) Climatic potential and on-farm yield trends of rice and wheat in the Indo- Gangetic plains. Field Crops. Res. 80: 223-234.

Pathak, H., Prasad, S. Arti Bhatia, Shalini Singh, S. Kumar, J. Singh, M.C. Jain (2003b) Methane emission from rice-wheat cropping system of India in relation to irrigation, farmyard manure and dicyandiamide application. Agric. Ecosys. Environ. 97: 309-316.

Paustian, K. (2002) Cropland management for carbon sequestration. www.colostate edu/Depts/Soil Crop/extension Newsletters/2002/May/May web/may09/html.

Paustian, K., Six, J., Elliott, E.T., Hunt, H.W., Rustad, L.E., Huntingdon, T.G. and Boone, R.D. (2000) Management options for reducing CO2 emissions from agricultural soils. Biogeochem. 48(1): 147-163.

Ponnamperuma, F.N. (1972) The chemistry of submerged soils. Adv. Agron. 24: 29-96.

Potter, C. S., Randerson, J. T., Field, C. B., Matson, P. A., Klooster, S. A. (1993) Terrestrial ecosystem production : a process model based on global satellite and surface data. Global Biogeochem. Cycles 7: 811-841.

Prade, K. and Trolldenier, G. (1988) Effect of wheat roots on denitrification at varying soil air-filled porosity and organic carbon content. Soil Biol. Biochem. 7: 1-6.

Prakasha Rao, E.V.S. and Puttanna, K. (1987) Nitrification and ammonia volatilization losses from urea and dicyandiamide treated urea in a sandy loam soil. Plant Soil 92: 201-206.

Prasad, R. and Power, J.F. (1995) Nitrification inhibitors for agriculture, health and the environment. Adv. Agron. 54: 233-281.

Prinn, R.G. (1995) Global atmospheric-biospheric chemistry. In Prinn, R.G. (Ed.) Global Atmospheric-Bioshperic Chemistry, Plenum, New York, 1-18 pp.

Prinn, R.G., Cunnold, R., Rasmussen, R., Simmonds, P., Alyea, F., Crawford, A., Fraser, P. and Resen, R. (1990) Atmospheric emissions and trends of nitrous oxide deduced from 10 years of ALE-GAGE data. J. Geophys. Res. 95: 18369-18385.

Rachpal-Singh and Nye, P.H. (1986) A model of ammonia volatilization from applied urea. III. Sensitivity analysis, mechanisms and applications. J. Soil Sci. 37: 31-40.

Radel, R.J., Randale, A.A. Gautney, J., Bock, B.R. and Williams, H.M. (1992) Thiophosphoryl triamide: A dual purpose urease/nitrification inhibitor. Fert. Res. 31: 275-280.

Rao D.L.N. and Pathak H. (1996) Ameliorative influence of Organic matter on biological activity of salt-affected soils. Arid Soil Res. Rehabilit. 10: 311-319.

Rastogi, M., Singh, S. and Pathak, H. (2002) Emission of carbon dioxide from soil. Curr. Sci. 82(5): 101-108.

Riley, W.J. and Matson, P.A. (1998) The NLOSS model. 1998 Fall AGU meeting. Poster A41B-25. AGU volume 79, Number 45, 10 Nov 1998.

Rodgers, G.A. (1983) Effect of DCD on ammonia volatilization from urea in soil. Fert. Res. 4: 361-367.

Rodhe, A.L. (1990) A comparison of the contribution of various gases to the greenhouse effect. Science 248: 1217-1219.

Roy, R., Klüber, H.D. and Conrad, R.F. (1997) Early initiation of methane production in anoxic soil despite the presence of oxidants. FEMS Microbiol. Ecol. 12: 311-320.

Ryan, J., Lal, R. (ed), Kimble, J.M., Follett, R. F. (ed) and Stewart, B.A. (1998) Changes on organic carbon in long term rotation and tillage trials in Northern Syria. Management of carbon sequestration in soil. 285-296 pp.

Saenjan, P. and Wada, H. (1990) Effects of salts on methane formation and sulphate reduction in submerged soil. In: Transactions 14th International Congress of Soil Science, Kyoto II, 244-247 pp.

Sarkar, M.C., Banerjee, N.K., Rana, D.S. and Uppal, K.S. (1991) Field measurements of ammonia volatilization losses of nitrogen from urea applied to wheat. Fert. News 36(11): 25-28.

Saseendran, S.A., Singh, K.K., Rathore, L.S., Singh, S.V., Sinha, S.K. (1999) Effects of climate change on rice production in the tropical humid climate of Kerala, India. Climatic Change 12:1-20

Scott, A., Ball, B.C., Crichton, I.J. and Aitken, M.N. (2000) Nitrous and Carbon dioxide emissions from grass land amended with sewage sludge. Soil Use Manage. 16(1): 36-41.

Setyanto, P., Makarim, A.K., Fagi, A.M., Wassmann, R. and Buendia, L.V. (2000) Crop management affecting methane emissions from irrigated and rainfed rice in Central Jawa (Indonesia). Nutr. Cycling Agroecosys. 58: 85-93.

Sharma, S.K., Kumar, V. and Singh, M. (1992) Effect of different factors on ammonia volatilization losses in soils. J. Indian Soc. Soil Sci. 40: 251-256.

Sihag, D. and Singh, J.P. (1997) Effect of organic materials on ammonia volatilization losses from urea under submerged condition. J. Indian Soc. Soil Sci. 45: 822-825.

Singh, J.S., Raghubanshi, A.S., Reddy, V.S., Singh, S. and Kashyap, A.K. (1998) Methane flux from irrigated paddy and dryland rice fields, and from seasonally dry tropical forest and savanna soils of India. Soil Biol. Biochem. 30: 135-139.

Singh, J.S., Singh, S., Raghubanshi, A.S., Singh, S. and Kashyap, A.K. (1996) Methane flux from rice/wheat agro-ecosystem as affected by crop phenology, fertilization and water level. Plant Soil. 183: 323-327.

Sinha, S.K. and Swaminathan, M.S. (1991) Deforestation, climate change and sustainable nutritional security: a case study of India. Climatic Change. 19: 201-209.

Sitaula, B.K., Bakken, L.R and Abrahamsen, G. (1995) N-fertilization and soil acidification effects on N_2O and CO_2 emission from temperate pine forest soil. Soil Biol. Biochem. 27(11): 1401-1408.

Skiba, U., Hargreaves, K.J., Beverland, I.J., Oneill, D.H., Fowler, D. and Moncrieff, J.B. (1996) Measurement of field scale N_2O emission fluxes from a wheat crop using micrometeorological techniques. Plant Soil. 181, 139-144.

Slattery, W. J. and Surapaneni, A. (2002) Can organic fertilizers enhance carbon sequestration in soils? 17th WCSS, 10th Symposium: Paper no.1705.

Smith, K.A. (1980) A model of the extent of anaerobic zones in aggregated soils and its potential application to estimates of denitrification. J. Soil Sci. 31: 263-277.

Sriegel, R.G., McConnaughey, T.A.,Thorsteson, D.C.,Weeks, E.P. and Woodward, J.C. (1992) Consumption of atmospheric methane by desert soils. Nature. 357: 145.

Stewart, B. A. (1993) Managing crop residue for the retention of carbon. Water, Air, and Soil Poll. 70: 373-380.

Swaminathan, M.S. (1995) Intensive farming: Rationale of integrated systems. In Hindu Survey of Indian Agriculture, 7-13 pp.

Teraguchi, S. and Hollocher, T. C. (1989) Purification and some characteristics of a cytochrome c-containing nitrous oxide reductase from *Wolonella succinogenes*. J. Biol. Chem. 264: 1972-1979.

Topp, E. and Knowles, R. (1984) Effects of nitrapyrin [2-chloro-6-(trichloromethyl)pyridine] on the obligate methanotroph (*Methylosinus trichosporium* OB3B). Appl. Environ. Microbiol. 47: 258-262.

Vilsmeier, K. (1991) Turnover of ^{15}N ammonium sulphate with dicyandiamide under aerobic and anaerobic soil conditions. Fert. Res. 29: 191-196.

Vlèk, P. L.G. and Henning, M. (1995) Fert. Res. 42: 165-174.

Wang, B. and Adachi, K. (2000) Differences among rice cultivars in root exudation, methane oxidation and populations of methanotophic and methanogenic bacteria in relation to methane emission. Nutr. Cycling Agroecosys. 58: 349-356.

Wang, B., Neue, H.U. and Samonte, H.P. (1997) Effect of cultivar difference ('IR72', 'IR65598' and 'Dular') on methane emission. Agric. Ecosys. Environ. 62: 31-40.

Wang, Z.P., De Laune, R.D., Masscheleyn, P.H. and Patrick, W.H. Jr. (1993) Soil Redox and pH Effects on methane production in a flooded rice field. Soil Sci. Soc. Am. J. 57: 382-385.

Wassmann, R., Buendia, L.V., Lantin, R.S., Bueno, C., Lubigan, L.A., Umali, A., Nocon,

N.N., Javellana, A.M. and Neue, H.U. (2000) Mechanism of crop management on methane emissions from rice fields in Los Banos, Philippines, Nutr. Cycl. Agroecosys. 58: 107-119.

Watson, R.T., Zinyowera, M.C., Moss, R.H. and Dokken, D.J. (1996) Climate change 1995, impacts, adaptations and mitigation of climate change: Scientific-technical analyses, Intergovernmental Panel on Climate Change, Cambridge University Press, USA, p. 879.

Whalen, S.C. and Reeburgh, W.S. (1990) Consumption of atmospheric methane by tundra soils. Nature 346: 160-162

Wilson, T.W., Webster, C.P., Goulding, K.W.T. and Powlson, D.S. (1995) Methane oxidation in temperate soils, Effects of land use and the chemical form of nitrogen fertilizer. Chemosphere 30: 539-546.

Yaduvanshi, N.P.S. (2001) Ammonium volatilization losses from integrated nutrient management in rice fields of alkali soils. J. Indian Soc. Soil Sci. 49: 276-280.

Yagi, K., Tsuruta, H. and Minami, K. (1997) Possible options for mitigating methane emission from rice cultivation. Nutr. Cycling Agroecosys. 49: 213-220.

Ying, Z., Boecky, P., Chen, G.X. and Van Cleemput, O. (2000) Influence of Azolla on methane emission from rice fields. Nutr. Cycling Agroecosys. 58: 321-326.

Yoshinari, T. (1990) Emissions of N_2O from various environments - the use of stable isotope composition of N_2O as tracer for the studies of N_2O biogeochemical cycling, In: (Eds) Revsbech, N.P. and Sorenson, J. Denitification in Soil and Sediment, 129-149 pp.

Zogg, G. P., Zak D. R., Ringelberg D. B., Mac Donald N.W., Pregitzer K.S. and White D.C. (1997). Compositional and functional shifts in microbial communities due to soil warming. Soil Sci. Soc. Am. J. 61: 475-481.

Subject Index

2-amino-4-chloro—6-methyl-pyrimidine (AM)   53, 107, 110
2-sulphanilamide-thiazole (ST)   110
Abiological reactions   34
Absorption band   18
Aceticlastic pathway   22
Acetylene   53
Acid rain   125
Acid soils   58
Acid trap method   73
Adaptation   117, 93
Advanced International Studies Unit (AISU)   117
Aerenchyma tissues   24
Aerosol   6
Air pollution   103
Agriculture   105
Albedo   125
Alliance of Small Island States (AOSIS)   126
Alcaligenes   81
Alternate wetting and drying cycles   37
Alternative energy   126
Aluminium carbide (Al_4C_3)   18
Ammonia (NH_3)   15, 56, 64
Ammonium nitrate   40, 60
Ammonium sulphate   29, 39, 59, 109
Anaerobic carbon mineralization   27
Anaerobic decomposition   126
Anaerobiosis   80, 99
Anhydrous ammonia   39, 40
Annual   10, 15, 19, 23, 52, 76
Antarctic "Ozone Hole"   126
Anthropogenic   34, 126
Assimilatory nitrate reduction   34, 36
ATC (4-Amino,1,2,4-triazale)   110

Atmosphere   24, 4
Atmosphere   126
Aquatic   9, 24, 50, 57, 93
Atmospheric abundance   34
Atmospheric pressure   52
Atom   9
Azolla   59

Bacteria   94
Band stretching   9
Baseline emissions   126
Berlin Mandate   126
Biodegradable   127
Biodiversity   97
Biofuel   14, 127
Biogas slurry   29
Biogeochemical Cycle   127
Biological nitrogen fixation   15
Biological oxygen demand (BOD)   40, 127
Biomass energy   127
Biosphere   127
Borehole   127
Bituminous coal   18
Blackbody radiations (Model)   2
Boiling point   18, 34
Bond   9
BOX_4 104
Brassica   89
Buffering capacity   60
Bulk density   66
Burning of biomass   5, 6

C: N   12, 17, 31, 81, 90, 101
C3 plants   10
Calcium nitrate   39

Carbon   96
Carbon cycle   127
Carbon dioxide (CO_2)   9, 10, 47, 96
Carbon dioxide equivalent (CDE)   7, 8, 12
Carbon equivalent (CE)   7, 8, 12
Carbon monoxide (CO)   15
Carbon reserves   48
Carbon sequestration   48, 55, 96, 105, 128
Carbon sinks   128
Carbon stock   49
Cation exchange capacity   60
CEC   60
CENTURY model   104, 44
Chapman reaction   7
Chemoautotrophic methanogens   22
Chemodenitrification   34
Chlorofluorocarbons (CFCs)   6, 128
Chlorophyll meter   108
Clay loam soil   39
Clayey soil   39
Climate   96, 129
Climate change   11, 12, 96-95, 129
Climate feedback   129
Climate lag   129
Climate model   129
Closed Chamber Method   65, 55-68
Coastal lands   12
Coated-fertilizers   60
Composting   129
Conference of Parties (COP)   129
Conservation buffer   102
Conservation tillage   99
Continuous flooding   16
Cowpea   61
Crop growth   12, 15, 32
Crop residue   100
Crop respiration   10
Crop rotations   100
Cropland   102
Crops   53
Cultivars   93, 29, 112
Cyanobacteria

DAISY   104
Deforestation   104, 130
Desertification   130
Degradation   31
Degraded land   102
Denitrification   33, 34-35, 53, 56, 81
Desertification   91, 87

Dicyandiamide (DCD)   53, 62, 107, 110
Diffusion   24, 27, 42
Direct crop establishment   16
Direct N_2O emission   76
Diseases   91
Dissimilatory nitrate reduction   34-36
Distillation   18
DMPP (3,4-Dimethyl pyrazole phosphate)   111
DNDC model   44, 104
Drought   1, 5, 10, 11
Dry seeded rice   16, 31

Earthworms   98, 55
Ebullition   24, 26, 42
Ecological systems   9
Ecosystem   24, 33, 56, 75, 79, 130
El Ninõ   11, 130
Electromagnetic spectrum   18
Electron acceptors   22, 27
Electron capture detector (ECD)   70
Emission   5, 15, 16, 18, 27, 32, 36, 46, 50, 55, 130
Emission inventory   75, 130
Emissions coefficient/factor   131
Encapsulated ECC   53
Energy   2, 11, 22
Enhanced greenhouse effect   56, 131
Environment   131
Environmental pollution   5
Evapo-transpiration   12

Fermentation   22
Fertilization, Carbon dioxide   131
Fertilizer formulations   64
Fertilizer placement   46, 107
Fertilizer tax   113
Fertilizers   29, 33, 39, 45, 53, 56, 57
Fertilizer-use efficiencies   11, 14, 33
Fisheries   9, 11
Flame ionization detector (FID)   69
Floods   10, 11
Fluorocarbons   131
Forcing Mechanism   131
Food security   11
Forestry   8, 9
Formaldehyde dehydrogenase   23
Formate dehydrogenase   23
Fossil fuel combustion   5, 6

Fugitive emissions   131

Gas chromatograph   69, 70
General Circulation Model (GCM)   2, 131
Global Environment Facility (GEF)   116
Global warming   2, 5, 15, 81, 131
Global Warming Potential (GWP)   67, 131
Grassland   102
Gravimetric soil water content   37
Green Revolution   5-6
Greenhouse Effect   2, 4, 5, 9, 47, 132
Greenhouse gas   57, 96, 132
Groundwater   86

Harvest index   16, 31
Heat balance   2
Homonuclear diatomic molecules   9
Human health   9
Humification-mineralization cycle   55
Hydrocarbon   18
Hydrochlorofluorocarbons (HCFCs)   132
Hydrofluorocarbons (HFCs)   132
Hydrogen
Hydrogenotrophic pathway   22
Hydrologic cycle   132
Hydrolysis   58
Hydroxyl amine   36

Immobilization   41
INC/FCCC   116
Indirect N_2O emission   77
Industrial emissions   5
Infrared radiation   3, 132
Intergovernmental Panel on Climate Change (IPCC)   9, 19, 115, 133
Internal motion   8
Inventory of GHG   13
Irrigation   64, 95, 111

Joint implementation   105, 133

Karanja seed extract   111
Kyoto Protocol   96, 105, 133

Landfill   134
Lifetime (Atmospheric)   134
Land-management   36
Land-use   45, 63, 112
Laughing gas   34

Leaching   34, 53, 56, 75, 77
Lignin   100
Liming   101
Long-chain polymers   97
Long-wave radiation   2, 4, 134

Maize   88
Manuring   97
Melting point   18
Methane (CH_4)   18, 134
Methane consumption   23
Methanobacterium   80
Methanogenesis   21, 22, 30, 80
Methanogens   21, 22
Methanotrophs   23, 80
Methanotropic   134
Methylococcccus capsulatus   80
Methylotrophic methanogens   22
Microaggregation   97
Micrometeorological Method   66
Microorganisms   23, 34, 80
Mid-season aeration   16, 31
Mid-season drainage   16, 30, 31
Mineralization   41
Ministry of Environment and Forests   21
Mitigation   30, 55, 106
Modelling   44, 104
Moisture   51, 83
Moisture regime   37, 40, 59
Molecular weight   34, 48
Monoxygenase   23
Methanol dehydrogenase   23
Monsoon   87
Montreal Protocol   134
Mount Pinatubo   134
Mulching   52

Nuse efficiency   106, 107
Natural gas   34, 18, 48, 135
Nature   18
NESWA Model   104
Nitrapyrin   31, 53
Nitric oxide   7
Nitrification   34, 62, 133
Nitrification inhibitors   53, 62, 107, 110-111, 113
Nitrite   34
Nitrobacter vulgaris   81
Nitrobacter winogradskyi   81
Nitrococcus mobilis   81

Nitrogen cycle 135
Nitrogen oxides (NO$_x$) 15, 135
Nitrosolobus multiformis 81
Nitrosomonas europaea 81
Nitrosovibrio tenuis 81
Nitrospira briensis 81
Nitrous oxide (N$_2$O) 5, 15, 56, 135
Nitrous oxide reductase 354
Non-respiratory N$_2$O producers 36
Northern Hemisphere 18
No-till agriculture
Nutrient management 101
Nutrient mineralization 11

OBM Model 104
Oceans 43
Open Chamber Method 65
Organic amendments 16, 28, 52
Organic manure 52
Organic matter amendment 61, 40
Oscillatory motion 9
Oxidative activity 16
Oxygen 38
Ozone (O$_3$) 7, 57, 135
Ozone depleting substance (ODS) 135
Ozone layer 5, 135
Ozone layer depletion 5, 56
Ozone precursors 135

Perfluorocarbons (PFCs) 136
Pests 91
pH 28, 38, 51, 59, 60, 66
Phosphogypsum 29
Photosynthesis 47
Phytoplanktons 5
Plant 41, 61, 82
Pollution 136
Pastures 103
Porosity 97
Precipitation 86
Productivity 87
Pseudomonas 81

Q$_{10}$ function 28, 82

Radiative forcing 136
Radioactive ^{63}Ni
Rainfall 59
Rangeland 103
Recycling 136
Renewable energy 136

Redox potential 22, 28, 38
Reduced tillage 93, 97
Relative humidity 66
Renewable energy 136
Residence time 136
Residue incorporation 97
Restoration 102
Rhizosphere 42
Rice 88
Root respiration 100
Root system 16
Run-off 56, 77, 99

Salinity 52
Salinization 102, 87
Salt tolerance 92
Salts 30
Sandy loam soil 53
Sea level 12
Sesbania 100
Short wave radiation 4
Single super phosphate (SSP) 29
Sink 136
Stratosphere 137
Sulphate aerosols 137
Site-specific integrated nutrient management system 64
Site-specific nutrient management 108
Sodium acetate 18
Sodium hydroxide 72
Sodium thiosulphate 53
Soil 96
Soil carbon content 97–99
Soil colloids 110
Soil conditioners 55
Soil depth 54
Soil erosion 15, 90, 102
Soil fertility 101
Soil organic matter (SOM) 83, 99
Soil organic matter 83, 90, 96
Soil processes 55
Soil respiration 51, 54, 71, 73
Soil texture 30, 39, 45, 51, 66
Soil water availability 90
Soil water-content 38, 41, 44, 50
Solar radiation 27
Sources 59
Southern Hemisphere 18
Sparingly soluble 18
Specific gravity 34

Split application 64
Stratospheric ozone 33
Sugarcane 88
Sulphate-containing fertilizers 29, 31
Summer Fallows 102

Temperature 27, 39, 50, 59, 61, 83
Tetrahedron 18
Thermophilic 39
Tillage 54, 93, 99, 112
Trace Gas 137
Troposphere 4, 5
Tropospheric O_3 20, 137

Ultraviolet light 5
Ultraviolet radiation (UV) 5, 137
United Nations Conference on Environment and Development (UNCED) 117
United Nations Conference on the Human Environment (UNCHE) 116
United Nations Environment Programe (UNEP) 116
United Nations Framework Convention on Climate Change (UNFCCC) 138
Urea 39, 40, 58
Urea inhibitor 107

Urea super-granules 59, 60
Urease enzyme 58
US Environmental Protection Agency

Vascular transport 24, 42
Vibrational motion 8
Volatilization 15, 56, 57–64
Vulnerability 90

Water 30, 31, 35, 39
Water management 30, 101
Water resources 86
Wavelength 2
Wax-coated calcium carbide 110
Weather 138
Weeds 99
Well-fermented manure 16
Wetland 102
Wheat 87
Wind speed 27, 42, 61
Wind velocity 90
Wollinella succinogenes 81
World Meterological Organization (WMO) 117

Yield gap 93

Author index

Adachi, K.   147
Adams, R.M.   2
Adamsen, A.P.S.   20
Adhya, T.K.   29
Aggarwal   87, 88
Allen   86
Anderson, I.C.   20, 139
Arah, J.R.M.   139
Aulakh, M.S.   101, 21

Baker   86
Baladioli, M.   44
Banerjee, B.   62, 11, 56
Batjes, N.H.   99
Battle, M.   140
Beauchamp, E.G.   140
Bhatia, A.   33
Bhattacharya, S.   140
Blake, D.R.   19
Blackmen   110
Bremmer, J.H.   110
Bundy, L.G.   140
Buresh, R.J.   140
Burton, D.L.   140
Buyanovsky, G.A.   51

Cai, Z.C.   29
Castaldi, S.   140
Cattle, H.   22, 2
Chaareonsi, N.   29
Chander   100
Cohen   92
Chatterjee, A.   88
Chattopadhayay, R.   89
Chaudhary, A.   79
Cicerone, R.J.   21
Conrad, R.   141

Dadhwal, V.K.   141
Davidson E.A.   44
De Datta, S.K.   141
Debnath, G.   29
Donner, L.   19
Doran   101
Duxbury, J. M.   109

Ehhalt, D.H.   18
Eichner, M.J.   40

Fenn, L.B.   141
Ferm, M.   141
Fillery, I.R.P.   61
Firestone M. K.   44

Galbally, I.E.   40
Garg, A.   13, 15
George, T.   142
Gorissen, A.   82
Govind, A.   115
Granli, T.   142
Gupta, P.K.   24
Gupta, Raj K.   49

Hargrove, W.L.   61
Heidt, L.E.   18
Hollocher, T. C.   81
Holzapfel-Pschorn, A.   2
Houghton, R.A.   47, 49
Hrtwig, U.A.   142
Hulme, C.J.   92
Hutchinson, G.L.   143
Hutsch, B.W.   143

Jain, M.C.   30
Jain, N.   18

Jyothi Kumari   115

Kalra, N.   87
Kicklighter, D.W.   49
King, G.M.   20
Kumar, S.   1, 18
Kumar, U.   143

Ladha, J.K.   143
Lal, R.   102, 143
Lessard, R.   144
Li, C. S.   44
Lu, W.F.   30
Lyster   60

Machida, T.   144
Majumdar, D.   40
Matson, P.A.   44
Mazumdar, S.   40, 56, 111
McConnaughey, P.K.   141
Migeotte, M.V.   18
Mishra, S.   144
Mitra, A.P.   24
Mitra, S.   18
Mosier, A.R.   7, 44, 49, 99, 110

Nedwell, D.B.   87, 111
Neue, H. U.   23
Nye, P.H.   146

Oremland, R.M.   22

Page, A.L.   145
Palmer, R.R.   145
Parashar, D.C.   63
Parkin, T.B.   145
Parton, W.J.   44
Pathak, H.   37, 45, 52, 87, 111
Paustian, K.   49
Ponnamperuma, F.N.   145
Potter, C. S.   44
Power, J.F.   110
Prade, K.   145
Prakasha Rao, E.V.S.   146
Prasad, R.   110
Prasad, S.   33
Prinn, R.G.   19
Puri, S.   79
Puttanna, K.   146

Radel, R.J.   62
Rai, H.K.   47
Ramanathan, V.   19

Rao, D.L.N.   49, 52
Rastogi, M.   52
Reeburgh, W.S.   83
Riley, W.J.   44
Rodgers, G.A.   146
Rodhe, A.L.   146
Roy, R.   28

Saenjan, P.   30
Sarkar, M.C.   146
Saseenlran   88
Sundquist   49
Scott, A.   52
Seiler, W.   28
Setyanto, P.   29
Sharma, A.   47
Sharma, V.   33, 106
Shetter, J.D.   21
Shukla, P.R.   13, 15
Sihag, D.   147
Singh, J.P.   147
Singh, J.S.   147
Singh, P.K.   106
Singh, R.   96
Sinha, S.K.   147
Sitaula, B.K.   52
Skiba, U.   147
Smith, K.A.   147
Soni, U.A.   86
Sriegel, R.G.   147
Swaminathan, M.S.

Teraguchi, S.   81
Topp, E.   147

Varade, S.B.
Vilsmeier, K.   147
Vlek, P. L.G.   59

Wada, H.   30
Wang, B.   21, 26, 28
Wang, Z.P.   21, 26, 28
Wassmann, R.   29
Watson, R.T.   10
Whalen, S.C.   148
Wilson, T.W.
Wu   102

Yaduvanshi, N.P.S.   148
Yagi, K.   28
Ying, Z.   29
Yoshinari, T.   148

Zogg, G. P.   83